Praise for *Asian S*

"I Enjoyed Food, Stay Full & yet I Lost Weight"

"I lost 9.6 lbs from Dec 12 to Jan 10. People couldn't believe it.They said "Nobody loses that kind of weight over the Christmas and New Year Holidays." Yes you do if you follow Linda Yo's weight loss method. I enjoyed food, stay full and yet I lost weight."

Ken Blanchard, co-author of One Minute Manager

"Your Program is the Gift that Keeps on Giving"

"Because of the way that you have taught me to eat, I am now no longer a slave to food. I can eat without guilt and enjoy what I eat knowing full well that I am now in control and not my appetite.

Because of you I look great and others have noticed my SLIM SELF. Again thank you for your SECRET."

Sandy Wallace, Las Vegas, Nevada

"Lost 25 Pounds & Never Feel Hungry"

"Your plan was the only one that ever worked for me. I've lost weight and I never feel hungry. It's magical!! Thank you so much for sharing your secret!!"

Patty McCormick, Ventura, CA

"We can Benefit by Expanding Our Knowledge of this Asian Cuisine"

"During our extensive experimental research for the China Study, I have come to realize that it is the kind of food, more than the amount of food, that is primarily responsible for all around health. The China Study shows that the Asian traditional diet is healthy; thus we can benefit by expanding our knowledge of this Asian cuisine."

T Colin Campbell, PhD, author of the China Study, Professor Emeritus of Nutritional Biochemistry at Cornell University

"I Don't Have to be Hungry and Miserable"

I love the Asian Slim plan. It hits the mark for me in key areas. First, I don't have to be hungry and miserable. I feel full and satisfied between meals. Second, I really prefer eating warm food to the cold food offered on most other food plans. Third, the portions are large even though the calories are low. Fourth, I'm not suffering cravings because there is a big variety of foods to choose from. Fifth, my husband can eat the same foods and he's happy too. Sixth, I'm consistantly losing weight, week after week and starting to exercise. Seventh, it's very interesting to learn to prepare Asian foods. I thought Asian cooking was too complicated to even try, but it is much easier and faster than I imagined

Frieda Barken, wife & assistant to Dr. Barken, San Diego, CA (to date Frieda has lost 100 lbs)

ASIAN SLIM SECRETS

LINDA YO, MS

*Nutritionist, Author, Speaker,
Personal Trainer, Health Coach*

AARONS MEDIA

AARONS MEDIA

www.AsianSlimSecret.com
info@AsianSlimSecret.com

SAN: 257-0742

Photographer: Brian Howarth

Dear Reader,

This book is dedicated to you.

I had been overweight and I know the pain. The journey to weight loss is not an easy one, especially when there are so many methods that deliver empty promises.

However, never, ever give up.

I have found a simple solution for enjoying food and staying slim, and you will too... if you keep on learning. So, take out your highlighter and start reading.

Best wishes,

Linda Yo

PS. You can find more resources at
www.AsianSlimSecret.com

When you give someone a book, you don't give him just paper, ink and glue. You give him the possibility of a whole new life.

Christoper Morley,
novelist, journalist and poet

Contents

Disclaimer

This book is written as a source of information only. The suggestion for specific foods and exercises in this book are not intended to replace appropriate and necessary medical care. If you have a medical condition please consult your physician. If any recommendation in this book contradicts your physician's advice, check with your doctor before you proceed.

Efforts have been made to make sure the information in this book is accurate. However, there may be mistakes, either typographical or in content. Therefore, this text should be use as a general guide only and not as the ultimate guide of health and exercise information.

The author and the publisher expressly disclaim any liability or loss resulting from the directions given in the book.

Acknowledgments

I thank God for allowing the pain of being overweight come to my life, for the joy of learning and for the revelation about the benefit of Asian eating habits.

I would like to thank the following terrific individuals: Barbara Beattie of Clear Copy Editing for her excellent services; Dr. Janine Higgins for being patient in answering my questions; Loanny Stankich for keeping the pictures I would never otherwise preserved; Judy Cullins for her guidance, Linda P. Smith, Charles (Chuck) Shockley and all the friends at the La Mesa writing class; Cathi Stevenson, Brian and Valerie Howarth, Valerie Fowler, Michael Hartanto for their artistic talent.

Last but not least, I thank my husband for his continuing patience, prayers and support.

About the Author

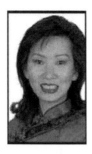

Linda Yo, MS gained twenty five pounds in three months when she moved from Asia to the U.S. She failed at every weight-loss method before finally getting results by returning to Asian eating habits.

Amazed by the results and because of her passion for good foods, she dedicated 28 years of her life to study and research the benefits of Asian eating habits.

Linda Yo, MS holds a master degree in nutitional sciences from San Diego State University. She combined the eastern philosophy of eating with modern science to discover the most effective way to lose weight and stay slim without dieting, pills or excessive exercise.

She is a passionate teacher and speaker in the area of weight loss and self development.

Linda Yo is available for speaking engagements, training seminars and private weight-loss coaching. Contact her at lindaasianslim@gmail.com.

The journey of a thousand mile begins with a single step.

Chinese Proverb

At Last, a Permanent Solution!

I was a skinny girl when I first came to the United States thirty years ago. But after several months of eating American food, I gained 25 pounds.

For two years, I fought to lose the weight. I read at least a dozen weight-loss books; I tried diet patches, fat reducing creams, diet pills, diet tea, Slim-Fast, and everything that was on commercials at the time. The expensive diet patches and fat-reducing creams showed no results even though I applied them religiously. The diet tea gave me diarrhea for a few days, and I lost a couple of pounds. Then it lost its power, and my stomach didn't react anymore. Consequently, I gained back the weight, most of which was probably water anyway. Slim-Fast was just like any regular milk for me. I would stay full for an hour, and then be hungry again. It could not substitute for a regular meal. Diet pills were a scary experience. They made my heart beat so fast, I thought it was going to explode. I also followed the directions in the many diet books I bought, but the result was always yo-yo weight loss; I would lose 5 pounds, then gain back 7 pounds. It was very discouraging.

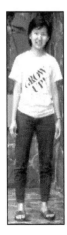

I began to reflect back on when I was growing up in Asia. I was a skinny girl with a big appetite. Meals would last for an hour and I usually ate two to three plates of food in addition to mid-morning and mid-afternoon snacks and also supper. I then began to realize that American food was the culprit.

Prior to coming to the US, I was slim.

My two girlfriends who are also from my country are good cooks. They cook and eat traditional food all the time. I always thought they had "skinny genes."

Whenever we went to the mall, they had fun trying on clothes. However, I could not find anything that looked good on me. Frustrated, I always ended up going to a bookstore to look for a new diet book to help me lose weight.

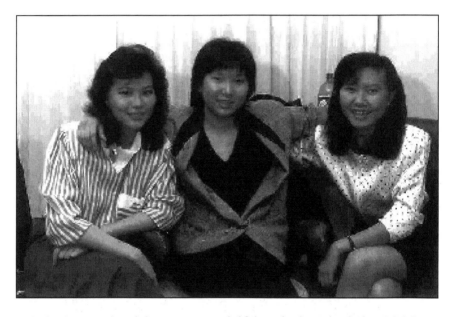

Me (center) with my two girlfriends in Virginia, 1988.

Compare this with my picture on the book cover and I think you will agree with me that 17 years later, even though I am growing older, I look a lot better. So read on...

After I reduced my intake of American food and prepared my food the traditional way, I lost the 25 pounds without hunger or deprivation.

When I went back to my country, I feasted every day on favorite foods that I cannot find in the United States. I ate at least three big meals and two to four snacks every day. I never gained weight at all.

Even throughout my pregnancy and my good life in a typical upper middle class family in Indonesia, I stayed slim. This was in spite of the fact that I was a stay-at-home mom with two live-in maids who did everything from taking care of the baby to shopping and cooking for my family.

I have traveled to Japan, Singapore, Hong Kong and Taiwan. These are developed countries in Asia where the standard of living is almost equal to the people in the United States. However, the people there are noticeably slimmer than the average American.

Since I love to eat, I observed and asked people lots of questions about their dietary habits. Their answers confirmed what I already suspected. The people who maintained their traditional diet stayed slim while the people who adopted western dietary habits gained extra weight.

I researched more on this subject by taking nutrition classes and joining the graduate program at San Diego State University specialized in nutritional sciences. All the good diets supported by the most respectable experts pointed to a diet similar to the Asian diet.

This book is a summary of what I have learned and practiced over the last 28 years. It is a practical, common sense guide on how to enjoy food and stay slim with minimal effort.

You don't even have to like Asian food to benefit from this book. A minor adjustment on how you enjoy your regular food can lead you to the path of becoming naturally slim just like the Asian population.

When you want to learn how to drive, you turn to the people who already know how to drive. So, when you want to learn how to enjoy good food and stay slim, why not turn to the billions of Asian people who enjoy great food and stay slim? It just makes sense.

When the student is ready

the teacher will appear...

(I hope you are ready!)

The Asian Passion for Good Food

If you travel to Asia or to a Chinatown in the United States, you will see that Asian people are obsessed with food. There are a lot of eateries and food markets selling everything under the sun.

In countries like India, Thailand and Indonesia, house-wives spend hours grinding spices in a mortar and pre-paring family meals. In Singapore, Hong Kong and Japan where the pace is faster, there are tens of thousands of eateries.

Martin Yan, the famous chef of the television series *Yan Can Cook,* shares in his book, *Asia,* his experience about the Singaporeans' passion for eating. His Singaporean friends always insist on a breakfast, mid-morning coffee break, lunch, afternoon tea and snack, serious dinner and another snack before bedtime. While they eat, they discuss their favorite dishes, their recent restaurant discoveries and where to eat next.

According to Martin, Singaporeans admit that they have three national passions: shopping, working, and eating. Martin thinks the first two passions are just excuses to get out of the house to eat.

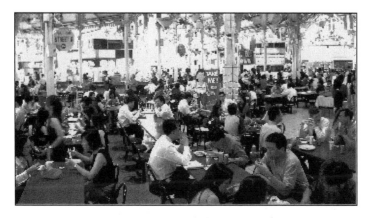

Singapore food court

After all, Singapore and many countries in Asia have the Chinese influence and the Chinese passion for food is reflected in their language and common expressions. The customary Chinese greeting when two friends meet is "Ni je fan le ma?" This means "Have you eaten rice/meal?" Eating with family and friends is our favorite activity. Birthdays, weddings and other celebrations are just more reasons for a ten-course meal.

The usual menu package at Chinese restaurants for this kind of occasion will include soup; various kinds of barbecue meat; chicken, beef or pork; tofu; vegetables, fish, shrimp or lobster dishes; fried rice or noodles; and will end with fresh fruit or sweets for dessert.

At home, warm meals are served three times a day, and they include rice or noodles with three to five dishes. Most Asians consume three to four pounds of food every day.

Yet, the people are slim!

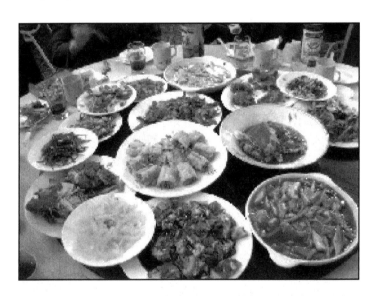

This picture was taken by Mrs. Anita DeFina, while attending a wedding reception in China.

The World Factbook published by CIA revealed that the rates of obesity in developed nations in Asia such as Japan, Singapore and South Korea in 2008 are less than 8%, very low when compared to the US where 33% of the population is obese.

A survey by CDC in the United States also shows that while the rates of obesity are high for the Latino, Black, and White populations, Asian Americans have a relatively low rate of obesity. Is it because of our genes? I know it is not, because I had gained weight easily when I ate American food and had to fight hard to lose it. Also, Asian children and teenagers who have changed their diet from traditional Asian food to burgers, hot dogs, pizzas and sodas are becoming obese at an alarming rate.

To lose weight, Americans should learn how the Asians eat. The Pritikin diet was very successful in the 1970s and helped many people to reverse their coronary artery disease by acknowledging this fact and encouraging people to eat complex carbohydrates, natural food and a low-fat diet. Unfortunately, what has stuck in people's minds is only the concept of low fat. Americans have realized that high fat is not good for them, but they continue to overindulge in simple carbohydrates (sugar) such as sweets, cookies, and soda.

In the same decade, the Atkins diet was introduced. This diet was not popular then but made a big comeback in the 90s. People were tired of counting calories and being on a highly restricted diet. They embraced this diet because it allowed them to eat high-fat foods. A survey shows that in 2004, about 80% of Americans who were dieting had tried either the Atkins or the South Beach Diet.

Yet, the rate of obesity keeps increasing. The American public is confused. Every day it seems there is a new opinion about how to lose weight. Nutrition issues become like political issues in that people take a stand in favor of or against them.

To benefit from this book, I ask you to proceed with an open mind. You are about to learn the diet of billions of people in Asia, the only continent in the 21st century where prosperity does not equal obesity.

Teachers open the door.

You enter by yourself.

Chinese Proverb

How Rice and Noodles Keep Asians Slim

Asians eat rice two to three times a day. In fact, steamed rice is a staple food and no meal is complete without it.

What about the low-carb diet advice to reduce the consumption of carbohydrates?

The low-carb diet is not a healthy way of life. For decades, many experts have warmed the public about low carb diets because:

1. In the long term, low carbohydrate diet will result in complications such as heart arrhythmias, cardiac contractile function impairment, sudden death, osteoporosis, kidney damage, increased cancer risk, impairment of physical activity and lipid abnormalities. (Bilsborough, 2003)

2. It goes against the recommendation of doctors and nutritionists from major organizations:

- The American Heart Association (2012): "doesn't recommend high-protein diets for weight loss...People who stay on these diets very long may not get enough vitamins and minerals and face other potential health risks."

- Australian Heart Foundation (2008): "the Heart Foundation does not support the adoption of very low carbohydrate diets for weight loss."

- Food Standards Agency of United Kingdom (2008): "rather than avoiding starchy foods, it's better to try and base your meals on them." They further state concerns regarding fat consumption in low-carbohydrate diets.

- Heart & Stroke Foundation of Canada (2012): "In a recent survey of Canadian dietitians, 97 percent said that choosing the right carbs is better for healthy eating than choosing a low-carb diet."

3. The use of protein for metabolism causes the secretion of toxic substances. The body draws a lot of water from its cells (which are 70% water) to flush these toxins. The rapid loss of water gives false promise of weight loss.

4. The presence of toxins and chemical imbalances caused by a high-protein diet results in bad breath, fatigue and headaches.

5. The diet lacks fiber, increasing the risk of constipation and colon disease.

What About the Glycemic Index?

The Glycemic Index (GI) measures how fast sugar from a certain food is absorbed into the bloodstream compared to white bread. The GI of white bread is 100. Other foods are compared to white bread to determine their GI score. The higher the GI, the faster sugar from the food is absorbed by the body.

A diet based on the Glycemic Index does not take into account the calorie count, the fat content and the volume of food.

Which is less fattening?

	GI	Calories	Fat (mg)
1 Snickers bar	57	280	14
or			
1 cup of carrots	70	45	0

1 cup of ice cream	87	400	20
or			
1 cup of baked potato	158	110	0

Proponents of a diet based on the Glycemic Index teach that foods with a low GI promote weight loss. In this case, they mistakenly suggest that a Snickers bar is less fattening than a cup of carrots and that a cup of ice cream is better for weight loss than a cup of plain baked potato.

A low GI does not mean low calories and does not necessarily mean the food is healthy. The Glycemic Index is not a reliable guide for weight loss.

A review of 23 clinical trials that examined low GI/GL diets and weight loss as the primary outcome found that these studies showed much inconsistency in their findings. While a few studies found significantly greater weight loss on the low GI/GL diets, most studies showed a non-significant trend that favored low GI/GL diets; suggesting that factors other than GI/GL may play a role. (Esfahani, 2011)

Statistics indicate that rice-eating nations have a low rate of obesity.

Rate of obesity in 2008
Countries where people rarely eat rice

United States	33%
UK	26.9%
Australia	26.8%

Rate of obesity in 2008
Asian countries where people eat 2 to 5 cups of rice every day

Japan	5 %
South Korea	7.7%
Singapore	7 %

Enjoy Rice, Asian Style

Do you think steamed rice tastes bland? If you do, you probably do not eat it the same way Asians do.

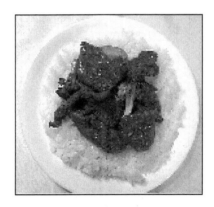

Steamed rice is a staple food in Asian cuisine. A plain baked potato tastes bland without a topping. Likewise, rice should be eaten with toppings of meat and vegetables.

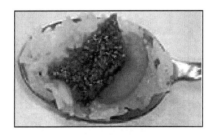

Eat rice with meat and vegetable dishes.
Put some rice, a piece of meat and vegetable on your spoon.

Rice is Not a Side Dish

If you think Asian food is too salty, spicy or sweet, maybe it is because you don't eat the dish with rice. Bland steamed rice is to complement and contrast the strong flavor of the dishes. Most Asian dishes are meant to be eaten with steamed rice.

If you want to add some flavor to your rice you can add low-calorie seasonings such as garlic salt, ginger, curry powder or chicken broth.

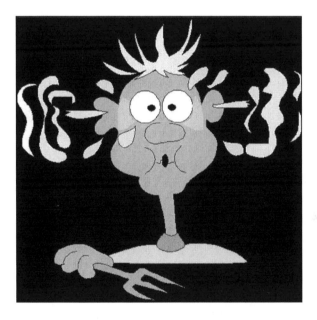

You are suppose to eat the Kung Pao kick with rice!

Eat Like an Asian: Increase Your Daily Intake of Rice

How rice keeps Asians slim:

Rice is bulky.
Rice is cooked with a lot of water. To make steamed rice you have to add 1½–2 cups of water for every cup of rice.

Comparison of Asian and Western Staple Food

Rice

Bread

Steamed rice contains 70% water; hence, it is large in volume but low in calories.

Bread is made up of a small amount of dough and lots of air. Air is lost in the chewing process. Bread enters the stomach as a small volume of food.

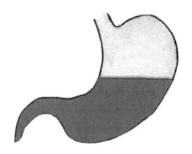 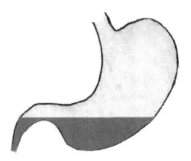

Because of the large volume, rice fills you up.

The smaller volume does not fill you up.

Your stomach can hold about 4–6 cups of food. The sooner your stomach is filled, the sooner it will send a message to the brain to stop eating.

Some people think rice is fattening because they feel stuffed after eating it. On the contrary, food with high water content such as rice, pasta and vegetables are large in volume but low in calories. This food supports weight loss because it fills you up, leaving you less prone to overeating.

Food that made you stuffed: High in water	IS NOT EQUAL TO	Food that made you fat: High in calories and fat

It's not the feeling that counts; it's the fat and calories. A candy bar or a piece of cheese is high in fat and calories but doesn't make you feel stuffed. This kind of food may cause you to end up eating even more to get that satisfied, full feeling.

According to Dr. Bell and Dr. Rolls (2001) in their study regarding the energy density of foods, cues related to the amount of food consumed have a greater influence on short-term intake than the amount of energy consumed.

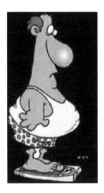

The best time to weigh yourself is early in the morning, after all the food from the day before is digested.

Are Carbohydrates Good or Bad for Our Bodies?

- Our bodies are always in need of carbohydrates as fuel for our activities.

- Our brains and nervous systems need carbohydrates to function properly.

For these reasons, trained athletes follow a diet high in carbohydrates.

If you look at the nutrition label on Gatorade or other sports drinks, you will find that they are high in carbohydrates. Our bodies need carbohydrates to function properly.

Let's take a close look at the Nutrition Facts of a 20 fl. oz. bottle of Gatorade:

Serving Size 8 fl. oz. (240 mL)
Serving Per Container 2.5

Amount Per Serving:
Calories 50

Total Fat 0 g
Sodium 110 mg
Potassium 30 mg
Total Carbohydrate 14 g
  Sugar 14 g
Protein 0 g

A 20 fl. oz. Gatorade will give you a total of 2.5 servings x 50 calories/serving = 125 calories. These 125 calories come from sugar (simple carbohydrate).

You burn a lot of carbohydrates when you exercise and sports drinks replenish them by supplying you with sugar which is a quick source of fuel and a simple carbohydrate.

There are 2 Kinds of Carbohydrates:

**Complex Carbohydrates
(Good Carbs)**

**Simple Carbohydrates
(Bad Carbs)**

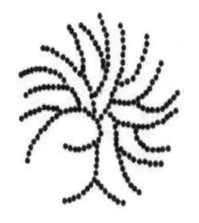

Complex structure, thousands of units strung together.

Simple structure, a unit stands alone or tied to one other unit.

Hard to digest: the stomach takes a long time to break down the complex structure; hence, they keep the stomach full for a long time.

Easy to digest: they quickly leave the stomach, making it empty and hungry again in a short time.

Found in: grains, beans, and vegetables.

Found in: sugar, honey, cakes, cookies and sweet drinks (including natural fruit juice).

Rice is a Good Carb

Experts at the USDA and the American Heart Association recommend that we consume plenty of grains every day because they are a good source of complex carbohydrates.

Complex carbohydrates (good carbs) take a long time to digest. They release the needed fuel slowly and steadily into the system, fulfilling the body's need without giving too much at a time, so there is no excess to be stored as fat. In contrast, simple carbohydrates (bad carbs) overflow a lot of sugar to the system at once and the system responds by storing some of it as fat.

Do you crave sugary snacks? Your body and brain might be telling you that you need carbohydrates. If you eat complex carbohydrates during meal time, you will experience fewer cravings for sugar.

Which is More Fattening, Carbohydrate or Fat?

Gram per gram, fat contains more calories than carbohydrate.

1 gram fat = 9 calories
1 gram carbohydrate = 4 calories

Our bodies convert all excess calories that we don't use to be stored as fat. The conversion process itself requires energy. However, it is easier for our bodies to store excess fats than excess carbohydrates.

- Fat from food and fat in the body are almost similar in form. Our bodies require only 3 calories to convert fat from food into our body fat. 100 calories from fatty food will give the body 97 calories to store.

- To convert 100 calories from carbohydrate into body fat, we need to expend 23 calories, leaving the body with only 77 calories to be stored.

For example :

1 tablespoon of mayonnaise (rich in fat):
100 calories, 11 g fat → gives us 97 calories to store

2 tablespoons of sugar (rich in carbohydrate):
100 calories, 0 g fat → gives us 77 calories to store

It is easier to get fat when you overeat fatty foods rather than sugar (carbohydrates).

Is Starchy Food Fattening?

A lot of people, even some experts, still think that starchy food is fattening. The Asian diet has been rich in starchy food for many centuries. In fact, starchy food is the key reason why Asians can enjoy a large amount of food and stay slim.

Surprising New Findings About Starchy Food

Resistant Starch

In the past, it was thought that all starch in food is digested and absorbed by the human body. However, current research has discovered that a significant portion of starch cannot be digested and will be expelled from our body. This portion of starch is called resistant starch.

This means our stomach will not digest this portion of starchy food, which will come out of the body as waste. What the stomach cannot digest, the stomach cannot absorb. So when we eat starchy food that contains resistant starch, we get a reduction of the calories!

Scientific Studies Reveal the Benefit of Resistant Starch

Behall & Howe (1995) showed that resistant starch only yields between 2-3 kilocalories/gram which is lower than typical carbohydrate that yields 4 kilocalories/gram.

Willis, Eldridge, Beiseigel, Thomas & Slavin (2009) compared the satiety response of resistant starch, corn bran, barley ß-glucan+oat fiber, polydextrose & low fiber food in a randomized, crossover study. On 5 separate occasions, fasted subjects completed 4 baseline visual analogue scales (VAS). Then they were fed 1 of 5 muffins which contains either: low fiber, corn bran, barley ß-glucan+oat fiber, RS & polydextrose. After that, additional satiety VAS was completed at 15, 30, 45, 60, 120, 180 minutes after baseline. Result shows that resistant starch and corn bran were consistently more satiating than low fiber food.

Bodinham, Frost and Robertson (2010) examined the effect of acute ingestion of resistant starch (RS) in reducing food intake in 20 young, healthy males. In an acute, randomized, single blind crossover study, the subjects were fed 48 g of RS and placebo. After eating identical meal & an overnight fast on 2 occasions (one week apart) they consumed either RS or placebo for breakfast & lunch. After 7 hours, they were fed a large ad-libitum meal. Results showed that supplementation with 48g RS significantly lowered energy intake at the ad libitum test meal compared to placebo.

Studies by Wilis et al. (2009) and Bodinham et al. (2010) showed that resistant starch positively influenced satiety and might be beneficial in reducing the obesity epidemic in human.

To get a clearer picture, we can see at how resistant starch affect obesity prone rats in the laboratory settings. Higgins et al. (2011) investigate whether resistant starch can attenuate weight regain on a high fat diet in rats. At first, they fed the rat ad libitum for 16 weeks then fed them a low fat diet to induce a 17% body weight loss. Then the weight reduced rats were maintained on an energy-restricted low fat diet for 18 weeks with or without a daily bout of treadmill exercise. Rats were then allowed free access to high calorie diet that contained either 0.3% or 5.9% levels of resistant starch and were relapsed to obesity and surpassed their original, obese weight.

They found that both exercise and RS reduced the percentage of lost weight that was regained over the 9 week relapse period. The combination of resistant starch &

exercise induced an effect greater than that of resistant starch alone.

Dietary resistant starch, with or without exercise, would be a beneficial component of a weight maintenance strategy following weight loss, even in the face of temporary periods of high fat consumption.

Eat Starch to Burn More Fat

A recent study at the University of Colorado Health Sciences Center led by Dr. Higgins, published in the October 2004 issue of *Nutrition and Metabolism*, found that the presence of 5.4% resistant starch in a meal increased the burning of fat in the body by 23%. And this increase is sustained throughout the day even if only one meal contains resistant starch.

This study shows that when resistant starch is present, our body changes the way it burns food: instead of burning carbohydrates, our body burns fat first, leaving little or no fat to be stored by our body.

This is a new finding, and many health providers and nutritionist still may not be aware of it.

The Asian people themselves may not know about this scientific finding. However, they have always enjoyed the benefit of a diet rich in starchy food: they stay full and stay slim!

Resistant Starch (RS) is found in the following foods:

• Processed starchy foods that have been cooked and served at room temperature or below, such as rice, noodles and pasta. Sushi rice and Basmati rice are especially high in RS.

• Legumes: beans and lentils. Legumes are very high in both RS and fiber.

• Whole grain cereals: oats, rye, wheat, corn.

• Seeds and nuts. But keep in mind that seeds and nuts are high in fat and calories.

• Food that has high amylose content such as Hi-Maize cornstarch.

• Unripe fruit, especially bananas.

• Starchy root vegetables such as potato, yam and yucca, if served at room temperature or below.

Cooking starchy food and serving them at room temperature or below increases the resistant starch (RS) content.

Perry's Story

Perry is a fast-food restaurant manager. Most of his co-workers have weight problems. He tells them to eat rice but they think rice is fattening.

While Perry eats lunch with the rice that he brings from home everyday, his co-workers tend to skip meals. Later, when they become hungry, they will grab "a snack" of french fries or a milkshake. Or they might eat salad with one or two packages of high-fat salad dressing. They don't realize that a large fries contains 540 calories, a milkshake has 580 calories, a small package of ranch dressing has 310 calories, and that all these things are very high in fat.

Perry, on the other hand, weighs only 150 pounds and has maintained this weight for many years. His secret? He eats plenty of rice as his staple food. He usually eats chicken nuggets or fried fish with a bowl of rice for lunch.

"Wait a minute! Aren't those fried things high in fat and calories?" you ask.

Yes, but if you enjoy these sinful pleasures with rice, you can still stay slim like Perry. Discover the secret on page 22, "Eat Starch to Burn More Fat," and on page 47, "How to Enjoy Fatty Food and Stay Slim."

Steamed Rice is Served Plain while Western Staple Food is Usually Served with Fats, Oils and Sugar

Bread by itself is low in fat, but the spread we put on it is usually high in calories and fat.

	Calories	Fat grams
1 tbsp. of butter	100	11
1 slice of cheese	110	9
1 tbsp. of margarine	100	11
1 tbsp. of cream cheese	50	5
1 tbsp. of mayonnaise	100	11
1 tbsp. of peanut butter	100	8

The USDA suggests that Americans limit their intake of total fat to 30% and saturated fat (generally fat from animal sources and dairy products) to 10% of their total calorie intake.

For example, if you are an active woman and your daily requirement is 2000 calories, you should limit saturated fat intake to 22 grams per day.

Rice will help you lose weight if you avoid or reduce the use of butter, margarine or oil while cooking it.

If you like flavored rice, try to use low-fat seasonings such as garlic salt, ginger, chicken broth or curry powder.

Types of Rice

- **White rice** is the most common rice used in Asia. The Chinese prefer long grain which is thin and dry, while the Japanese like short grain which is softer and slightly sticky. The long grain is best if used for fried rice while the short grain is best for sushi.

  Instant rice is white rice that has been precooked and dried. It is convenient but less tasty.

- **Brown rice** is the whole grain because it still retains its bran and germ. For this reason it has more fiber, vitamins and minerals. It has a nutty flavor and is chewier than white rice. This is actually the healthiest kind of rice. If you have diabetes and are concerned that white rice will raise your blood sugar, check with your doctor. Many doctors in Asia recommend brown rice to their diabetic patients.

- **Converted rice** is a trademark of Uncle Ben's. It is pressure-steamed before the milling process to force the nutrients from the bran layer to enter the rice.

- **White glutinous/sticky rice** tastes sweet and often is used to make snacks and desserts. Black glutinous rice has a sweet and nutty flavor.

- **Wild rice** is not actually rice but the seed of an aquatic grass, yet it has all the goodness of rice.

- **Jasmine rice** is long grain aromatic rice. This kind of rice is usually served in an upscale Chinese restaurant. Many large supermarket chains sell this rice.

- **Basmati rice** is long grain aromatic rice. It has a nutty flavor and is sold in some health food stores. Basmati rice can help you to lose weight faster due to its high resistant starch content.

Selecting and Storing Rice

- Long or short grain white rice is commonly available at the local supermarket, either in bulk or pre-packaged. Brown rice becomes rancid sooner than white rice so always check the "use by" date, or if you are buying in bulk make sure that there is no evidence of moisture.

- White rice can be kept in a cool dry place. If kept in an airtight container, it will stay fresh for a year.

- Brown, red and black rice should be kept in an airtight container in the refrigerator to stay fresh for six months.

Cooking Rice

To rinse or not
If you use imported rice or rice sold in bulk, rinse it to remove any impurities from the mill or the store. On the other hand, some prepackaged rice produced in the United States has added vitamins so rinsing it might remove the added nutrients.

Cooking rice in a pot or a pan
Most rice sold in packages comes with cooking instructions. Follow the instructions carefully to make perfect steamed rice. If there are no instructions, follow these steps:

White rice
Put 1 cup of white rice with 1½ cup of water in a pot. Cook on high heat, uncovered, until it boils. Stir gently. Cover tightly with the lid. Cook on medium-low heat for 15 minutes. Do not open the lid or stir during this time.

Brown rice
Put 1 cup of brown rice with 2 cups of water in a pot. Cook on high heat, uncovered, until the water boils. Stir gently. Cover tightly with the lid. Cook on medium-low heat for 40 minutes.

Cooking rice with a rice cooker
If available, follow the directions in the user manual.

In many Asian homes, a rice cooker is used for convenience. Just put in the rice and water, press the cook button and forget about it. It is pre-programmed to switch from high heat to low once the rice has boiled. It keeps the rice warm in case a family member is late for dinner. Rice cookers sell for about $15–$40 at Wal-Mart, Target or other major department stores. If available, buy the one with a nonstick frame inside because it's easier to clean.

Asian cooks use this rule of thumb for cooking with a rice cooker:

White rice
Put rice in the rice cooker and add water until the water level is about ¾ inch (first knuckle of the index finger) above the rice. Press the cook button and in 20 minutes the button will move to keep warm mode and the rice is ready.

Brown rice
Use more water than white rice. The water level should be about 1¼ inches above the rice. Press the cook button and it will be ready in 40 minutes.

Troubleshooting When Cooking Rice

- The water has been absorbed, but the rice is not cooked.
  Reasons: This type of rice requires more water, the heat was too high or the lid was not tight.
  Solution: Sprinkle 3–5 tablespoons of water, cover and cook in medium-low heat for 5 more minutes.

- The rice is cooked and tender, but there is excess water.
  Reasons: The type of rice requires less water, or you put too much water to begin with.
  Solution: Pour off excess water, then cook the rice uncovered until the water dries.

Reheating Leftover Rice

- You can keep leftover rice covered in the refrigerator for up to five days.

- To heat it, use a microwave oven or a pot. As a rule of thumb, use one minute of high heat in the microwave for one bowl of rice. If the rice appears dry, sprinkle some water on top before you heat it up.

- Cold, dry leftover rice is a perfect ingredient for fried rice. For a fat-free comfort food on a cold day, use the leftover rice to make rice porridge. Recipes are in Chapter 12.

Noodles are also a Popular Staple Food in Asia

Noodle soup is a common breakfast and snack in Asian countries.

Why are noodles (or pasta) good for you?

• They are an excellent source of complex carbohydrates (good carbs). Like rice, they provide a crucial energy source for our brain and body cells. Eating noodles may alleviate our body cravings for high-calorie sweets.

• When cooked, they absorb a lot of water. The water content of noodles or pasta is 70%, about the same as steamed rice. Noodles and pasta are bulky so they fill us up.

• They are rich in B vitamins, niacin and iron.

• They contain resistant starch which goes thru our stomach and small intestine undigested.

In Asia, noodles are comfort foods, usually eaten with soup. Another alternative is to stir-fry them with 1 or 2 tablespoons of oil, which does increase the calorie content. However, fried noodles are usually eaten with thinly sliced meats and lots of vegetables, making it overall a healthy low-calorie meal.

Noodles and pasta are good for you as long as you prepare them as the Asians do. Avoid or reduce oily and creamy sauces. Try the recipes in Chapter 12 and you will have a satisfying, low-fat meal or snack.

Varieties of Asian Noodles

- **Fresh noodles** are made of wheat flour, eggs, salt and water. They come in three shapes: thick (Shanghai style), thin and wide. They are perfect for stir-fry, soup or cooked with a sauce. For Hong Kong-style pan-fried noodles use the thin ones.

- **Dried wheat flour noodles** are made of the same ingredients as fresh noodles and taste about the same. Cooking time is slightly longer than the fresh noodles.

- **Rice flour noodles.** There are two kinds of rice flour noodles: the wider type used by the Vietnamese for their famous beef noodle soup and the thin ones which are more popular as rice sticks or rice vermicelli. Rice vermicelli has made its way to the local supermarket. The wider type, the Vietnamese "pho," is available fresh or dried in the Asian market. Either type can be used for Pad Thai, the famous dish of noodles with peanut sauce from Thailand. You will find both recipes in Chapter 12.

- **Mung bean flour noodles (bean threads)** are made from the starch of mung bean, the same legume that produces bean sprouts.

- The Japanese udon is made of wheat flour, salt and water. It is increasingly available in local supermarkets in the cold food section, packaged like the instant noodles and comes with a soup base mix.

Cooking Asian Noodles

- Follow the instructions on the packaging carefully. Most Asian noodles are softer than pasta and can be easily overcooked and become mushy.

- Always boil the water first.

- Drop the noodles in the boiling water.

- Add a teaspoon of salt if you like.

- Stir the noodles with a fork or chopstick to prevent them from sticking together.

- Don't add oil to the water because oil will coat the noodles and make them repel rather than absorb the sauce.

- Be careful not to overcook noodles. Most Asian noodles only require a few seconds to a few minutes of cooking. Fresh noodles cook faster. Fresh thin egg noodles cook in only ten seconds in boiling water.

- Test whether the noodles are cooked by lifting one strand and cutting it. It should be pliable and the color and the consistency in the middle and the side should be the same.

- Do not leave the noodles in hot water because it will cause them to be overcooked. Rinse the noodles with cold water and drain to stop the cooking process.

- Cover the noodles if you don't use them right away to prevent dryness. Rinse again before use to separate the strands.

Incorporating Rice and Noodles into Your American Plate

Some of the items below are high in fat and calories. However, if you eat them with rice, you will stay slim as discussed previously and also on page 45, "How to Enjoy Fatty Food and Stay Slim."

• Rice with sliced steak

• Rice with beef stew

• Ham and scrambled egg fried rice

• Rice and chicken or fish nuggets

• Rice and chili

• Noodles and sliced turkey

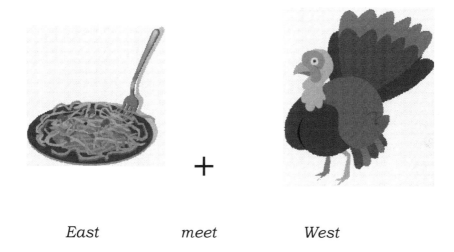

East   meet   West

= *Yum! + healthy*

Cut off this reminder and put it on of your refrigerator.

Build up Slimming Habits

• **Buy and store rice, noodles and pasta at home.**

• **Know how to cook steamed rice.**

• **Eat rice, noodles or pasta at least five times a week.**

• **Get a rice cooker to save time.**

4
Appetizers That Soothe Your Hunger

In Asia, appetizers are usually warm soups. Our stomachs quickly recognize the soup as a warm meal. As we empty our bowls, our stomachs are about ¼ full.

Asian-style soup is very light in calories. Asian people enjoy clear soups as well as thick ones. In Chinese homes, clear soup is often served as a drink and enjoyed throughout the meal.

The clear soup is similar to American chicken noodle soup; Asians are just more creative with the ingredients. Broccoli, cauliflower, carrots, mushrooms, squash, beans, shrimp or tofu can be added. This kind of soup is healthy and satisfying but low in calories and fat.

We use cornstarch instead of cream or milk to thicken our soups. Cornstarch is a complex carbohydrate (good carb) that has zero fat.

Compare the Soups

Thickened with Cornstarch
Size: 1 cup

Thickened with Cream
Size: 1 cup

Asian-Style Corn Soup
93 calories
   1 gram fat

Cream of Broccoli Soup
200 calories
   12 grams fat

Crabmeat and Asparagus Soup
74 calories
   2 grams fat

Clam Chowder Soup
240 calories
   15 grams fat

You can eliminate 520 calories, 60 grams of fat and 200 milligrams of cholesterol in your favorite soup and still achieve the same thickness just by replacing a cup of cream with two tablespoons of cornstarch. Or, if you like the taste of cream, you can use ¼ or ½ cup of cream instead of a whole cup and still eliminate a lot of calories and fat.

If you use evaporated fat free milk instead of cream, you will eliminate 380 calories and all the fat and cholesterol per cup.

You can find cornstarch in your local supermarket, usually in the baking section.

Directions: Always mix cornstarch well with a few tablespoons of cold water before use to prevent lumps in your soup.

Do Our Stomachs Treat Soup Like Water?

Our stomachs treat warm soup differently from water. Cold water leaves the stomach quickly. That is why we don't stay full just by drinking water. Warm liquid stays longer, especially when we add high-fiber, unprocessed vegetables in the soup.

An experiment in the 1980s by Henry Jordan, M.D., at the University of Pennsylvania involved 500 people in a weight loss program. These people were instructed to eat soup at least four times a week and to record every meal they ate for 10 weeks. The people who ate more soup ate fewer calories overall and lost more weight compared to those who ate soup less frequently.

A study by Zhu & Hollis in 2013 revealed that people in the US rarely consume soup. In winter months, about 60% of US adults consume soup less than once a week and this number goes up to 80% during other seasons.

The study indicated that soup consumption was associated with a lower BMI and waist circumference, as well as a reduced risk of being overweight or obese in the US adults.

A study by . Bertrais et al (2001)in France found heavy soup consumers (5-6 times per week) are slimmer (have a higher frequency of BMI <23 kg/m2) compare to occa-sional and non soup consumer (have a higher frequency of BMI>27 kg/m2).

In Portugal, Moreira and Padrao (2005) found that there is an association between soup consumption and body weight in Portuguese men and women suggesting a reduced risk of obesity in soup consumers.

In Japan, the median sup consumption was 7 times per week which indicated over half of the population was daily soup consumers. A study by Kuroda et al. (2011) found that the frequency of soup intake have a significant inverse association with BMI, waist circumference, and waist-to-hip ratio. and overall the obesity rate in Japan was very low.

Although all these studies occur in different countries, there is a consistent result suggesting the inverse association between soup consumption and body weight.

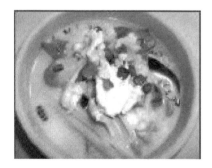

Warm, delicious & filling!

Soup and Rice as a Meal for Easy Weight Loss

When I met my husband, he was a little chubby by Asian standards. He was 175 lbs at 5 feet 7 inches. He and I love to eat so I never bothered him about his weight. After all, extra weight was a sign of prosperity in Indonesia.

In 1995, he received bad news from his doctor. His cholesterol level was 280. His doctor told him: "Lose 25 pounds or you will have to depend on prescription drugs for the rest of your life."

My husband lamented to me, "I have been 175 lbs for as long as I can remember. There is no way I can get down to 150 lbs!"

At the time, he worked at the head office of KFC-Indonesia. His office was just above the restaurant. He ate fried chicken and fries for lunch three to five times a week.

I asked him to switch from his regular lunch to rice and chicken soup. Fortunately, KFC in Indonesia served two kinds of chicken soup: chicken and vegetable clear soup and chicken with corn chowder, thickened with cornstarch.

Once or twice a week when he had cravings, he would still enjoy a piece of fried chicken and a small fries with his rice and soup lunch. In only twenty weeks, he reached his target weight and his cholesterol level dropped to 200 (normal) without him ever feeling extra hunger or taking any medications.

Twenty years later, my husband at age 56 still weighs 150 pounds, wears size 31 pants and looked better than the day I met him. (Of course, with the help of hair regrowth treatment he got from Costco!)

Soup Diet

Have you heard about the Cabbage Soup Diet? This diet was once popular. One of my ex co-workers is a true believer since she always lost weight with it.

There is only one problem. She is fed up eating the same soup day in and day out. I suggested to her to make the same kind of clear soup and be creative with the ingredients. As long as you use vegetables, reduce or skip the meat and cream, you have a healthy meal.

Chicken, beef or vegetable broth or bouillon and spices such as ginger, garlic and varieties of Asian seasonings I describe in Chapter 8, give rich flavors and are low in calories. Use varieties of fresh, frozen or canned vegetables with grains or beans to avoid boredom.

Vegetables cook in a short time and taste best when they are still a little crunchy, so pay attention to the cooking time to prevent an overcooked and mushy taste.

I suggest you eat vegetable soup and rice instead of salad if you want to lose weight fast because:

- Warm soup is more filling than cold salad.

- Most salad dressings are very high in calories and fats. A small package of two ounces of ranch dressing contains 310 calories and 33 grams of fat! In many restaurants some salads contain as many calories as large burgers.

- A combination of vegetables or beans and rice gives your body the essential proteins.

Why Doesn't the Starvation Diet Work?

Many of us have tried fasting or skipping meals and we know that it doesn't work.

When we fast, our bodies think we are starving. The body then tries to conserve energy by slowing down its metabolism. Slower metabolism means the body burns less energy during daily activities. This is why people on prolonged fasting will hit a plateau in their weight loss.

When we return to our normal eating patterns, it takes a while for our bodies to adjust from the slower metabolism to our regular metabolism. During the adjustment period, we will have surplus calories which our bodies store as fat.

What Works?

Experts agree that the best diet plan is to reduce calorie intake by a small amount, about 500–1000 calories, every day. Since one pound is equal to 3500 calories, you will lose 1–2 pounds a week or 4–8 pounds a month

----

Studies show that the people who lose weight slowly with a healthy diet are more likely to maintain their healthy weight for a long term.

In my husband's case, he did not even feel like he was on a diet. He simply replaced his usual high-calorie, high-fat lunch with a low-fat soup and rice lunch. When he had cravings, after he ate his rice and soup, he ate a small portion of the high-calorie food. Since he was always full and satisfied, he did not think of food all the time like most dieters.

Build up Slimming Habits

- **Enjoy soup as your appetizers or snacks.**

  Rice + Soup = Full Stomach + Calm Soul + Slim Body

Quick Soup Ideas

- Canned vegetable soups such as corn, lentil, chicken and vegetable soup are low in calories and fat. Chicken noodle soup is also a healthy choice and goes well with rice. Heat them up with rice in the microwave and you have a warm and satisfying meal.

- Any kind of vegetable--fresh, frozen or canned--tastes great with chicken-flavored soup. If you add ginger and minced garlic or garlic salt, they will taste delicious.

- Use instant noodles and replace the high fat seasoning with one cube chicken or beef bouillon and ¼ teaspoon salt and pepper. Add vegetables and salad shrimps or an egg white to make a satisfying, low-calorie meal.

- Make a scrambled egg; add water, vegetables and garlic salt and you have a nutritious soup in five minutes.

In Chapter 12 you will find favorite soup recipes from Hong Kong, Japan, Indonesia, Thailand, and Vietnam.

When you buy soup, canned or from a deli, make sure to check the calories and fat content. Avoid American-style creamy soups since heavy creams are used as thickeners and they are very high in calories and fats.

How to Enjoy Meat and Avoid the Fat.

Some people think that Asians don't eat meat on a daily basis. That might be true for the people who live in rural areas of some developing countries. But most Asians who live in the cities, especially in developed countries like Singapore, Japan, South Korea and also here in the US, enjoy meat every day.

The difference between Asian and Western meat dishes is in the method of preparation of the meat.

Asian Method of Cooking Meat

The meat is sliced into thin pieces.

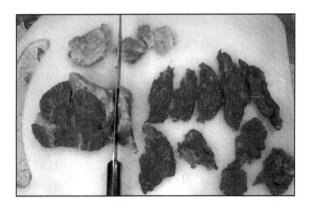

All the visible fat is easily discarded.

The sliced meat can better absorb the seasoning.

As a result, the meat has a strong flavor, saltier or spicier.

Because of the strong flavor, it has to be eaten with something bland such as steamed rice.

Varieties of vegetables are added to give color and contrast and to complement the meat dishes.

Western Method of Cooking Meat

Big, thick slices.

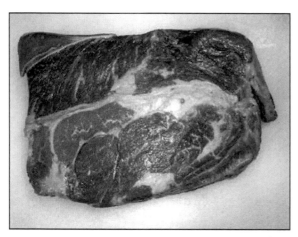

A lot of fat (marble) is trapped inside the meat.

Because of the thickness, it does not absorb the seasoning well. It has a weak, blander flavor compared to Asian meat dishes.

To add more flavor, butter, cheese or meat sauce is added.

Typically served with potatoes or bread with additional oil and fats.

Vegetables are served on the side, usually with high-calorie, high-fat dressings.

If you enjoy meat the Asian way, you will find it easy to adhere to the recommendation by the American Heart Association to eat no more than 6 ounces of lean meat in a day (about the size of two decks of cards).

Why do Scientists Suggest that Americans Limit Their Daily Intake of Meat?

- It is high in cholesterol.

- It is high in saturated fat. Scientists found that other than the natural cholesterol found in food, our body produces cholesterol from the saturated fat we consume. Since meat is high in both cholesterol and saturated fat, it gives us double trouble.

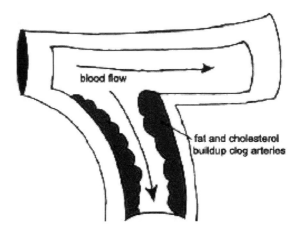

Fat and cholesterol form a buildup which clogs the arteries and blocks the flow of blood, which leads to hypertension, stroke or heart attack.

- The low carb diet has been very popular, however, findings from controlled trials do not support its effectiveness compared to other conventional diets beyond 12 months (Dansinger et al, 2005 and Foster, 2003). Moreover complications such as heart arrhythmias, cardiac contractile function impairment, sudden death, osteoporosis, kidney damage, increased cancer risk, impairment of physical activity and lipid abnormalities can all be linked to long-term restriction of carbohydrates in the diet (Bilsborough, 2003)

All Fats are Not Created Equal

There are 3 kinds of fat:

- **Saturated fat** is bad because it raises cholesterol, which clogs up arteries.

  Characteristic: solid at room temperature
  Mostly found in meat and dairy products such as cheese, butter and cream.

- **Trans fat** is an unsaturated fat from vegetable oil, processed to become solid. It also increases cholesterol. Margarine is an example. Liquid or soft margarines contain less trans fat than the hard ones.

Limit your daily intake of saturated and trans fat to 10 % of your total calories (about 20 grams for most people).

- **Unsaturated fat**
  Unsaturated fat is not as bad as saturated fat. This kind of fat does not clog arteries but it is still high in calories (1 gram of fat yields 9 calories). When you eat nuts or use vegetable oil (including olive oil), keep in mind that they are very dense in calories.

  1 cup of peanuts = 840 calories
  1 tablespoon of vegetable oil = 120 calories.

  Characteristic: not solid at room temperature.
  Usually found in nuts, vegetable oil and fish.

Limit your daily intake of unsaturated fat to 20 % of your total calories (about 40 grams for most people).

How to Enjoy Fatty Food and Stay Slim

My family also loves American food, especially fried chicken and barbecued ribs. Once a week, we visit our favorite restaurant, and since they don't serve steamed rice, they let us bring our own. I figure as long as we enjoy these high-fat American fares with our steamed rice, we maintain a reasonable calorie density.

What is Calorie Density?

Calorie density measures and compares the amount of calories in a certain volume of food.

- **1 cup chicken noodle soup:**
  100 calories, 2 g fat
  Not dense in calories

- **1 cup peanuts:**
  840 calories, 71 g fat
  Very dense in calories

Our stomach has a finite size, about 4 to 6 cups. Suppose you really like peanuts and you eat 4 cups. That totals to 3360 calories. A healthier option is to eat 3 cups of chicken noodle soup first and then enjoy 1 cup of peanuts. This way you can still enjoy your favorite snack, stay full and reduce your intake by 2220 calories.

By combining high- and low-calorie foods, you significantly reduce your calorie intake. If you use this principle, you will be able to enjoy fatty foods and stay slim.

How to Balance Your Calorie Density Intake

Happy and Healthy Stomach
Balanced Calorie Density

	Calories	Fat(g)
2 pcs fried chicken	530	36
1 cup of rice	200	0.5
1 corn on the cob	75	1.5
1 cup fresh fruit	60	0
Total	865	38

Greasy and Unhealthy Stomach
High Calorie Density

	Calories	Fat(g)
2 pcs fried chicken	530	36
1 biscuit	190	10
½ cup coleslaw	190	11
1 slice pecan pie	480	21
Total	1390	78

Calorie Density – Rule of Thumb

• Food rich in water such as rice, noodles, soups, vegetables and fruits have low calorie densities.

• Fried foods generally triple or quadruple the calorie density of food. For example, a 3-oz potato contains 65 calories and 0 gram of fat, but a 3-oz small fries contains 265 calories and 15 grams of fat.

• Processed foods are very high in calorie density. Continuing the example above, a 3-oz potato chip contains 450 calories and 30 grams of fat.

• Red meats and dairy products (other than nonfat or low-fat products) have high calorie densities.

Balance the calorie density of your food and you will stay slim for life.

Asian Restaurant Secret to Tender Meat

How to cut

- Always cut across the grain

- It is easier to slice the meat thinly if you partially freeze it.

To tenderize

- Soak the sliced meat in a bowl with ½ teaspoon of baking soda for every pound of meat for 10–20 minutes.

- Rinse the meat and it is ready to use for cooking.

Choose Your Meat Wisely

Get leaner cuts: Look for the word "loin" or "round" in beef and pork

	Approximate fat %
• **Beef (lean cuts)**	
Top round, eye of round	30%
Round tip	36%
Tenderloin, sirloin	38%
• **Pork**	
Center loin pork chop/roast	26%
Tenderloin	26%
Top loin	36%
• **Poultry (white meat without skin)**	
Turkey	19%
Chicken	23%

Avoid fatty cuts and dark meats

	Approximate fat %
• **Beef (fatty cuts)**	
Brisket	48%–75%
Chuck blade roast	72%
Flank steak	51%–58%
Porterhouse steak	44%–64%
Ribs	75%
T-bone steak	68%
• **Pork**	
Bacon	40%–90%
Loin blade steak	50%
Ribs	54%
Shoulder blade steak	51%
• **Poultry (dark meat with skin)**	
Turkey with skin	47%
Chicken with skin	56%

Build Up Slimming Habits

• **Enjoy your meat as the Asians do:**

> • **slice the meat into thin or bite-size pieces**

> • **add vegetables**

> • **eat it with rice**

• **Buy a lower fat cut: Look for the word "loin" or "round" in beef and pork: top round, eye of round, round tip, tenderloin, sirloin.**

• **Poultry: Choose skinless white meat which contains about 50% less fat than dark meat with skin.**

6
High in Protein, Low in Fat

Fish

Most Asians love fish and eat it at least once a week. The Japanese like to eat sushi, fresh raw seafood and rice. In other parts of Asia, fish is steamed, grilled, stir-fried or deep-fried. Low-calorie seasonings and condiments are added to enhance the flavor and to create variety of seafood dishes.

Health Benefits of Fish

Low in fat
Fish provides as much protein as other meat but is very low in fat. It contains less than 5% fat, compared to most meat, which contains 25–75% fat.

Reduces your risk of heart disease and stroke
Fish contains essential omega-3 fatty acids. Your body can't make omega-3 fatty acid (a good fat); you can only get it from your diet. It is called a good fat because even though it is a type of fat, it helps to reduce the risk of heart disease by preventing blood clotting in the arteries.

In Greenland, the consumption of fish is high among the Inuit people. It has been observed that even though their diet is high in fat and cholesterol, the incidence of coronary heart disease is low.

The American Heart Association recommends that we consume at least 2 servings of baked or grilled fish each week.

Reduces your risk of Alzheimer's disease

Omega-3 fatty acids are also needed by the brain's synaptic membranes (connections between brain cells) which are believed to help the brain to think more clearly.

A seven-year study on 815 nursing home residents found those who ate fish at least once a week had a 60% lower risk of Alzheimer's compared to those who seldom or never ate fish.

Lowers blood pressure, reduces inflammation, protects against diabetes

Research also indicates that omega-3 fatty acids may help lower the blood pressure of patients with hypertension; reduce inflammation associated with rheumatoid arthritis, asthma, multiple sclerosis, and psoriasis; and help protect against diabetes.

High in vitamins and minerals

Seafood is rich in calcium, which is needed for healthy bones and teeth; niacin, which is essential for healthy skin; and vitamin B complex, which is needed for metabolic processes. Seafood also contains iodine, which is essential for the function of the thyroid gland; iron for the formation of red cells; and zinc, which speeds up the healing of wounds.

In Japan and Iceland where fish consumption is high, life expectancies are among the longest in the world.

Is it Safe to Eat Fish?

In 2004, the FDA and EPA issued a joint consumer advisory to inform pregnant woman, woman who intend to become pregnant, nursing mothers and parents of young children on how to get benefits from consuming fish and minimizing their exposure to mercury.

Key points of the advisory

- Fish and shellfish are an important part of a healthy diet because they contain high quality protein, omega-3 fatty acids and are low in saturated fat. A balanced diet that includes fish and shellfish can contribute to heart health and children's proper growth and development.

- For most people, the risk of mercury exposure from eating fish is not a health concern. However, an unborn baby or young children may be harmed by the levels of mercury in certain fish and shellfish.

Therefore, the FDA and EPA are advising women who might become pregnant, pregnant women, nursing mothers, and young children to avoid certain types of fish. It states:

1. Do not eat shark, swordfish, king mackerel, or tilefish because they contain high levels of mercury.

2. Eat up to 12 ounces (2 average meals) a week of a variety of fish and shellfish that are lower in mercury.

    - Five of the most commonly eaten fish that are low in mercury are shrimp, canned light tuna, salmon, pollock, and catfish.

- Another commonly eaten fish, albacore ("white") tuna has more mercury than canned light tuna. So, when choosing your two meals of fish and shellfish, you may eat up to 6 ounces (one average meal) of albacore tuna per week.

3. Check local advisories about the safety of fish caught by family and friends in your local lakes, rivers, and coastal areas. If no advice is available, eat up to 6 ounces (one average meal) per week of fish you catch from local waters, but don't consume any other fish during that week.

Follow these same recommendations when feeding fish and shellfish to your young child, but serve smaller portions.

(Source: http://www.epa.gov/waterscience/fishadvice/advice.html)

How to Cook Fish

You will find great fish recipes in Chapter 12. Some fish are more suitable than others for a certain method of cooking. You can use tuna and salmon for any cooking method.

- **Sushi:** Very fresh sea bass, tuna, salmon fillets

- **Steamed (Chinese style) or poached:** bass, red snapper, halibut, cod, trout.

- **Grilled:** sea bass, red snapper, bonito, tilapia, yellow tail, salmon, pompano, permit.

- **Stir-fry:** any boneless fish fillet is great for stir-frying.

- **Boiled with sauces:** sea bass, red snapper, halibut, cod

- **Deep-fry:** any kind of fish is suitable for deep frying. Marinade fish with lemon juice or vinegar and a generous amount of salt for 15 minutes before frying. To reduce the splashing of oil, sprinkle some cornstarch on the fish before you drop it in the hot oil.

Use lime juice or vinegar to get rid of the fishy smell.

Shrimp

Many people avoid shrimp because of the cholesterol content. Fifteen large shrimps contain about 200 milligrams of cholesterol, almost equal to an egg yolk.

Nevertheless, studies show that eating shrimp raises LDL (bad cholesterol) by 7% but at the same time also raises HDL (good cholesterol) by 12%, making shrimp an overall healthy food.

Shrimp is rich in omega-3 fatty acids that are noted for their benefit in preventing heart disease, stroke, Alzheimer's disease and many other diseases.

Shrimp is low in calories and fat. Three ounces of cooked shrimp contain only 90 calories and 1.5 grams of fat, making it an ideal food for those who want to lose weight.

Asians cook shrimp in various ways. I always have a bag of peeled shrimp in my freezer because they are quick to thaw. Just dip them in a bowl of water and they are ready for use in a few minutes. They are a wonderful meat substitute or as an addition to fried rice, fried noodles, and soups, as well as meat and vegetable dishes.

How to Select and Store Seafood

• Look for shiny skin and bright eyes with black pupils. The body should be firm.

• Seafood is very sensitive to temperature and will spoil easily. Fish and shrimp last in the refrigerator up to two days. If you freeze them, you can extend their shelf life up to one month.

- Most fish in local supermarkets is already scaled and cleaned. In Asian supermarkets, we give directions to the fishmonger as to whether we want him to clean (gut), scale or cut the fish. Some places have fryers and will fry the fish at no additional cost.

- The best way to defrost seafood is to place it in a bowl of water or put it in the refrigerator for several hours.

How to Prepare Shrimp

Depending on the recipe, shrimp can be cooked either shelled or unshelled.

If you want to save time, buy unshelled and deveined shrimp.

To unshell shrimp
Pull off the head and peel the shell. When you reach the tail, hold the body and pull away the tail.

To devein shrimp
Cut the back of shrimp with a scissors and use a toothpick to pull out the black vein.

Tofu

Tofu is a custard-like food, made from soybean. It has a bland flavor by itself, almost like a plain potato. The condiments that we cook with the tofu gave it taste. Tofu goes well with curry sauce, peanut sauce, oyster sauce and many more Asian sauces. It is also combined with meat or vegetables to contrast and complement the tofu's fine texture.

It is high in protein but very low in calories and fat. A 3-oz serving size contains only 70 calories and 3 grams of fat. Tofu has many health benefits:

Prevents heart disease
Research shows that eating soy protein can lower your blood cholesterol level and reduce your risk of heart disease.

Lowers your risk of breast, prostate and uterine cancer
Soy contains isoflavones, which are believed to lower incidence of cancer. In countries like Japan where soy consumption is high, the incidence of breast, prostate and uterine cancer is among the lowest in the world.

Prevents osteoporosis
Tofu is rich in both calcium and isoflavones, making it a natural alternative to hormone replacement therapy. It reduces the risk of osteoporosis. A study showed that compared to Caucasian women, Asian women, though they consume less milk, have a lower incidence of hip fracture.

There are Many Kinds of Tofu

- **Soft and silken tofu** tastes very smooth and silky-soft. It is perfect for soup. You can also fry it but because of its soft nature, it may not stay together. Use silken tofu for miso soup and reduced-fat cheesecake.

- **Extra firm and firm tofu** are almost as firm as a cooked potato. They are perfect for frying. You can also use them for soup but generally soft tofu tastes better. Most Chinese and South East Asia dishes use firm tofu.

- **Pressed tofu** is firmer than the extra firm tofu. Usually it is seasoned and salted. Use it for salads or stir fry dishes. The Chinese like to eat this salted tofu with their porridge in the morning. Pressed tofu lasts up to 2 weeks in the refrigerator

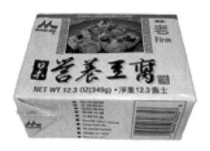

Japanese style tofu

Shopping

You can find tofu in the refrigerated section in the super-market. Often it is in the "health food' or "organic" area of the refrigerated section. Some Japanese tofus don't need to be refrigerated and are sold in the Asian food section of the supermarket.

Storing

An open package of tofu can be stored in the refrigerator up to five days provided it is covered with water and the water is changed daily.

Preparation

Drain the liquid in the tofu box if you purchase the kind that is soaking in water. The water has no nutritional value.

Cooking

Using a sharp knife, slice the tofu block into several strips. Pile the strips together and slice them into ½ inch cubes. The tofu is then ready for cooking. Cooking time for tofu is approximately 2–5 minutes depending on the firmness. Soft tofu requires less cooking time than firm tofu.

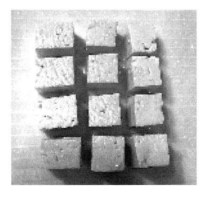

Tofu cubes

Build Up Slimming Habits

- **Eat seafood twice a week.**
Many supermarkets sell frozen fish and shrimp. You can also keep fresh seafood in the freezer until you are ready to use it. Try some new recipes from Chapter 12. A quick way to enjoy fish is to marinade it with salt and lime juice, grill it and eat it with low-fat condiments such as soy or chili sauce or salsa. See the recipe for seasoned soy sauce and tomato sauce condiments in Chapter 12.

- **Add tofu to your soup or your regular dishes.**

Tofu Ideas

- Beef and tofu chili

- Chicken, tofu and noodle soup

- Beef, tofu and vegetable stew

- Stir-fried tofu and ground meat (Mapo tofu, recipe in Chapter 12)

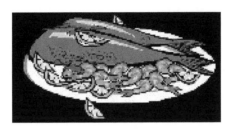

Seafood is high in protein, low in fat and calories and it has many health benefits.

7
The Best Food for Weight Loss

Everyone knows that vegetables are healthy. Yet, the American way of serving them may not be so healthy.

Comparison between Asian and American Vegetable Dishes

Mixed Vegetables Stir-Fry (Chinese Style)

94 calories
 4 grams fat

Small Caesar Salad With Dressings

360 calories
 26 grams fat

Asian vegetable dishes are very low in calories and fat. Yet they are tasty, warm and filling.

The method of preparation is quite simple. Most Asian vegetable dishes can be prepared in 15 minutes. The secret to a delicious vegetable dish is the perfect cooking time. The vegetables should still be crunchy and sweet and their color vibrant. Because of the short cooking time, most of the important vitamins and nutrients are retained.

Asian recipes offer you various ways to enjoy vegetables. From the simple stir-fry with garlic to the use of various sauces such as soy, oyster, curry or bean, Asian vegetable dishes are not only delicious but will help you lose weight.

Why are Vegetables so Beneficial?

If you are serious about losing weight, vegetables are your best allies for the following reasons:

1. Vegetables are high in fiber. Fiber is the part of plant food that our stomachs cannot digest.

   • Food with high fiber content takes a long time to digest, so it stays in the stomach and keeps you full for a long time.

   • Fiber helps prevent constipation, irritable bowel syndrome and colon cancer.

   • Fiber helps lower cholesterol. It binds with bile acids, the source of cholesterol, and brings them out of your body, thus helping to prevent heart disease.

2. Vegetables are large in volume but very low in calories. Compare a large amount of cauliflower with a small piece of cheese:

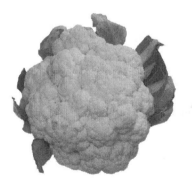

1 oz. cheese   4 cups cauliflower
110 calories   100 calories

3. Vegetables are rich in vitamins, minerals and phytochemicals. Phytochemicals are natural substances abundant in plant foods which are believed to prevent certain cancers and heart disease.

Fiber Keeps You Full and Makes You Slim

Fiber rich foods

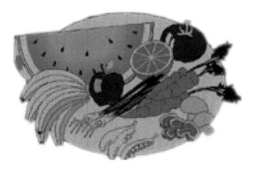

Fiber absorbs a lot of water. It's bulky and filling.
It is hard to process so it stays in the stomach for
a long time.

The stomach cannot process nor absorb the calories
from fiber. Fiber (and the calories it contains) will come
out of the body as waste.

Restroom

Free resources: www.asianslimsecrets.com

Various Asian Vegetables

To add variety and excitement to your plate, try Asian vegetables available in your local supermarket. These fresh, canned or dried vegetables are easy to use.

Bean Sprouts. They should look crisp and bright white. Brownish colors are a sign of staleness. Some Asian cooks insist on cutting the roots (which is done by hand). However, the roots are edible and it is okay to eat them. Rinse the bean sprouts thoroughly before use, but do not rinse if you are not using them right away. They will last up to 3 days in the refrigerator.

Bok Choy is a cabbage-like Asian green vegetable. It has white stalks and green leaves. A smaller one, called baby bok choy, is sweeter and softer than the regular bok choy.

Shiitake Mushrooms are available both fresh and dried. The dried ones have a fragrant aroma and taste better, but you have to soak them in hot water for 30 minutes before use.

Straw Mushrooms sold in cans in many local supermarkets. Rinse well before use to flush the "canned" taste.

Snow Peas or Chinese Peas are available fresh in local supermarkets. Cut both ends before use.

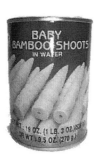

Young Bamboo Shoots. They are crunchy and sold precooked in cans in local supermarkets. Boil them for a minute, then rinse with cold water to get rid of the can taste. Some Asian markets also carry fresh ones. Always served them cooked because they are poisonous if eaten raw.

Water Chestnuts are available in local markets both fresh and canned. They taste sweet and crunchy. The Chinese believe they have yin properties or cooling effects and help relieve sore throat and fever.

Cooking Time for Fresh Vegetables

Each vegetable has a different cooking time. Pay special attention to this fact. When you stir-fry several kinds of vegetables in a pan or wok, drop in the ones with longer cooking time first, then the ones with shorter cooking time.

Longer cooking time (15 minutes)
Potatoes
Squash
Yams
Dried Shiitake Mushrooms

Medium cooking time (5–10 minutes)
Asparagus
Carrots
Celery
Eggplant
Green beans
Brussels sprouts
Lima beans
Kale
Zucchini

Short cooking time (2–5 minutes)
Bean sprouts
Bok choy
Corn
Mushrooms
Snow peas
Spinach & most green leafy vegetables
Most frozen or canned vegetables

How to Cut Vegetables for Stir Fry

Just like cooking meat, Asians cut their vegetables so they can easily absorb the condiments and cook quickly.

Here are illustrations on how to cut your vegetables the Asian way:

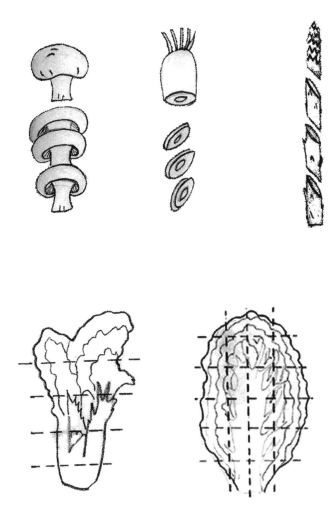

Secrets to Perfect Stir-Frying

1. Get all the ingredients ready. Read the entire recipe before you start. Slice the meat and the vegetables. Marinade the meat if needed. Premix the sauces. Put them near the pan or wok. Once you turn on the heat, there is no stopping. You have to be ready to drop the ingredients and stir continuously so the food cooks evenly.

2. Use a nonstick pan to reduce the need for oil. Heat the pan for a minute before you coat with a little oil or cooking spray. After the oil is hot (about 15 seconds) add the ingredients. Remember to turn on the exhaust fan so your house won't smell like a restaurant.

3. Know the cooking time of each vegetable and herb to decide which ones to add first, second and last. Generally aromatic seasonings such as onion, garlic and ginger will go first; then meat, poultry, seafood and vegetables in the longer or medium cooking time list. Leafy vegetables are usually the last be dropped in the pan.

4. Keep stirring and avoid overcrowding the pan or wok to ensure all the ingredients are evenly cooked.

5. Reduce the heat to low; taste and adjust the seasonings if needed before serving.

Build Up Slimming Habits

- **Keep plenty of frozen and canned vegetables at home.** They won't spoil easily and are available any time you need them. Thanks to today's technology, most vitamins and nutrients are preserved.

- **Be creative in adding vegetables to your meal:**

  - Add peas and carrots to stew and stir-fry dishes.

  - Shredded carrots, bean sprouts, chopped green beans or peas go well with omelets.

  - Corn is a great companion to any meal. Just heat it up in the microwave or stir-fry with garlic (and chili sauce if you like) to spice it up. Cook it with salad shrimps and you have a warm dish ready in five minutes.

- **You can use the microwave to steam vegetables.** Cooking time is about 1–3 minutes. Add oyster sauce or your favorite sauce and you have a warm vegetable dish.

- **Always have a jar of minced garlic and a bottle of soy sauce at hand.** You can prepare a quick vegetable stir-fry or soup with them.

- **Learn about Asian herbs, sauces and spices in the next chapter** so you can prepare a large variety of delicious, low-fat vegetable dishes.

8

Rich in Flavor, Low in Calories

Asian Sauces and Condiments

Most Asian sauces and condiments are made from plant sources and are thickened with cornstarch. Cornstarch is a complex carbohydrate (good carb) that is low in calories and fat. Compared to most western sauces, which are made from dairy products, Asian sauces are very low in fat and calories.

Comparison of Asian and Western Sauces and Condiments

Asian Sauces and Condiments	Western Sauces and Condiments
Soy Sauce, 1 tbsp. 10 calories, 0 gram fat	Ranch dipping sauce, 1 tbsp. 45 calories, 3 grams fat
Sweet and Sour Sauce, 1 tbsp. 20 calories, 0.5 gram fat	Tartar Sauce, 1 tbsp. 70 calories, 7 grams fat
Teriyaki Sauce, 1 tbsp. 15 calories, 0 gram fat	Mayonnaise, 1 tbsp. 100 calories, 11 grams fat

Many Asian sauces are sold in local supermarkets. You don't need to buy all of them to begin cooking Asian-style. For starters, buy two or three condiments and experiment with them until you feel more comfortable cooking Asian dishes.

The Following are the Most Widely Used Asian Sauces

Soy sauce: made from soybeans, wheat flour and brine. It may be used as salt replacement in some Chinese recipes. There are 2 main types:

- **Light soy sauce** ("light" is usually specified on the label). It is light in color, saltier and has a stronger flavor; best for stir-frying.

- **Dark soy sauce** (usually labeled as "soy sauce" only). This type has added caramel, is darker in color and milder than the light soy sauce. It is great for stewing or dipping sauce.

Most supermarkets carry dark soy sauce. Some also sell low-sodium soy sauce.

Oyster Sauce: made from cooked oysters, sugar, salt, caramel, wheat flour and cornstarch. It is used widely in Chinese cooking, is great for stir-fried meat or vegetables and can also be used as a soup base.

Chili sauce: made from red chili peppers, garlic, vinegar, sugar and salt. There are several combinations of chili sauce and the name will usually indicate the ingredients. Sweet chili sauce has added sugar. Garlic chili sauce includes more garlic than the regular ones. It is used for cooking as well as a condiment.

Rice wine: made from fermented glutinous rice. It tastes slightly sweet and has a flowery flavor.
To substitute: You can use dry pale sherry.

Sesame oil: made from toasted white sesame seeds. A small amount will add a nutty taste to the dish.

Teriyaki sauce: made from soy sauce, rice wine, brown sugar, ginger, garlic and pineapple juice. It has a sweet flavor and tastes great with barbecued or grilled meat, poultry and fish.

Black bean sauce: made from salted black beans and rice wine. Hot bean sauce is a combination of black beans and chili sauce. It is used with stir-fried meat, seafood, tofu or vegetables.

Fish sauce: made from fish extract. It adds a pungent aroma and slightly salty taste to soup or stir-fry dishes.

Curry sauce: made of curry powder, coconut milk and cornstarch solution. It goes well with all kinds of meat and vegetables.

Sweet and sour sauce: made of catsup, vinegar, sugar and cornstarch solution.

Rice vinegar: made from fermented rice. It is milder and sweeter than white vinegar.
To substitute: white vinegar.

Hoi sin sauce: made from fermented soybeans, garlic, vinegar, sugar and spices. It has a spicy and sweet flavor. It is used for cooking as well as condiment.

Peanut (sate) sauce: made from ground peanuts, shallots, garlic and coriander. It is used as a condiment to sate (grilled meat in skewer) and as a dressing for Indonesian salad.

Kung pao sauce: a combination of chilies, soybeans, ginger, garlic, sesame oil, sweet potato and other spices. It is used to create spicy dishes.

Coconut milk: made from coconut and is used in South East Asian recipes for curries, stews and dessert. An exception from the other Asian sauces, coconut milk is high in calories and saturated fat.

Shrimp paste: made from salted fermented small fish or shrimp. It has a strong pungent flavor. It is also known as "bagoon" in the Philippines, "petis" in Indonesia, and there is a dried version of the paste known as "blachan" in Malaysia.

Wasabi paste: a hot Japanese horseradish used as a condiment for sushi.

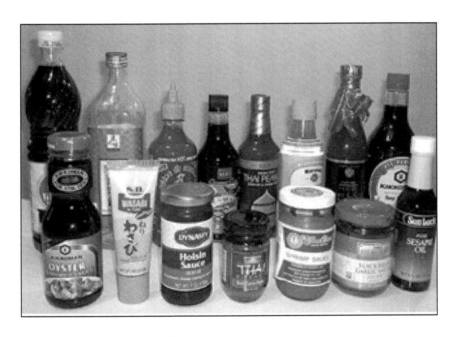

Front row (left to right): oyster sauce, wasabi paste, hoi sin sauce, curry sauce, shrimp sauce, black bean sauce, sesame oil.

Back row (left to right): fish sauce, rice wine, chili sauce, teriyaki sauce, peanut sauce, rice vinegar, sweet and sour sauce, soy sauce.

Are the Sauces High in Salt?

Some Asian sauces are high in salt content. However, because of the strong flavor, only a small amount of sauce is used. The use of these sauces also replaces or reduces table salt in the recipe. When cooking with Asian sauces, always taste before you add salt.

Is the Asian Diet High in Salt?

If you eat an Asian diet, you are more likely to eat less salt or sodium compared to your regular American diet.

- Asians eat vegetable and meat dishes with rice. Rice contains no sodium.

Staple Food	Sodium in mg
Rice	0
2 pieces of whole wheat bread	270

- Asian dishes rarely use processed meat and cheese which are high in salt.

Western Food	Sodium in mg
Turkey breast lunch meat, 2 oz.	500
Ham, 2 oz.	600
Cheese, 2 oz.	800

- In Asian homes and restaurants, salt shakers are rarely used in the dining room. The cook balances salt and other seasonings to the point of perfection in the kitchen. Adding salt is an insult to the cook. Never, ever use the salt shaker if the cook is your mother-in-law!

Fragrant Herbs and Spices

Herbs and spices add a lot of flavor and a negligible amount of calories. The most common herbs used in Asian cooking are ginger, garlic and green onions (scallions). All are rich in health benefits.

Ginger is an essential ingredient in soup or stir-fried dishes. Asian herbalists use ginger to treat stomach-aches and colds, cure drunkenness and stimulate circulation. Traditionally new mothers are given chicken soup with ginger to aid their recovery.

Ginger is available in many local supermarkets and can be stored up to two weeks in the refrigerator. It may last up to three months in the freezer.

To use: Rinse and peel the skin. Slice, mince or grate it according to the recipe or always grate it if you don't want to risk biting a piece of ginger which is quite spicy.

Garlic. For many centuries, garlic has been used as a medicine and flavoring agent in many parts of the world. Recent research shows that garlic is effective against some bacteria. It also reduces blood sugar, fats and high blood pressure.

The rule of thumb for using garlic in recipes is 1 clove is equal to 1 teaspoon of garlic.

Green onions (scallions) and onions are used to give flavor to fried rice or noodles, stir-fried dishes and soups. Throughout both the East and the West, onion has a reputation for being a home remedy for a huge range of illnesses including anemia, bronchitis, asthma, arthritis and loss of hair. Recent research indicates that consuming onions may reduce the level of blood cholesterol.

Start off your Asian cooking with the three most important ingredients: ginger, garlic and onions. When you are becoming more proficient, you may want to try new recipes with more exotic herbs and spices.

Chili peppers: Asians like to use small red chili peppers but actually you can use any kind of pepper to cook Asian cuisine. Generally small chilies are spicier than the big ones. Wash your hands after handling chili to avoid irritation to your skin or eyes.

Lemon grass: Sold fresh by the stalk in Asian markets, it has a subtle lemon flavor. It is also sold shredded and dried and needs to be soaked in hot water for 30 minutes before use.
To substitute: Use zest (the grated yellow peel) of a lemon. 1 tablespoon of zest replaces 1 stalk of lemon grass.

Star anise: Looks exactly like a star and it has a strong flavor.
To substitute: use anise seed or a cinnamon stick.

Coriander powder: Made from the seed of cilantro, it has a light sweet flavor. You can usually find it in your local supermarket. Some health food stores sell them in bulk.

Cumin powder: Made from aromatic seeds, it adds a pungent and mild flavor. Just like coriander, you might find them in your local supermarket.
To substitute: use caraway, but only a third of the amount of cumin needed in the recipe.

Galangal: A relative of ginger, it has a slight lemon and spicy mustard flavor.

Turmeric powder: Turmeric, another relative of ginger, has a pungent flavor. But if you overuse it, the dish will be bitter.

Kaffir lime leaves: Available in Asian markets, it is used heavily in Thai food.

To substitute: use citrus leaves.

Curry powder: A mix of turmeric, coriander seeds, cumin, chili peppers, cloves and cinnamon powders. Curry paste or sauce contains the same ingredients and usually tastes better than the powder. It is a ready-made ingredient for curry dishes.

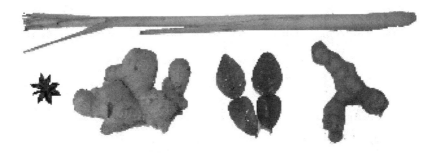

Back row: lemon grass

Front row (left to right): star anise, ginger, kaffir lime leaves, galangal.

Build Up Slimming Habits

- **Stock up on Asian sauces and herbs.**
For starters, get soy and oyster sauces, ginger, minced garlic and onion.

You can freeze most Asian herbs. Just soak them in water when you are ready to use them.

- **Check out the recipes in Chapter 12 and choose five of them.** Make a shopping list of the sauces, herbs and spices needed.

- **Always read the nutrition labels of your sauces.** Choose fat-free or low-fat sauces and condiments.

Choose
- Asian-style sauces and condiments
- BBQ sauce
- Mustard
- Ketchup
- Seafood cocktail sauce
- Salsa
- Steak sauce
- Tabasco or hot sauces
- Pasta sauces (if not mixed with cream or cheese)

Avoid or reduce
- Alfredo sauce
- Bearnaise sauce
- Mayonnaise
- Ranch sauce
- Tartar sauce
- Sour cream
- Sauces, condiments and salad dressings that contain cream or cheese.

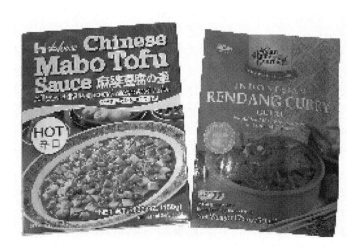

*Too tired to mince the herbs? Use
instant seasonings.*

9
Healthy and Delicious Snacks and Desserts

Fruits are the Asian people's favorite food for desserts and snacks. We value them as an important part of our diet. To the Indonesian, fruit is a "cuci mulut" which translates as "mouthwash." Fruits are believed to clean the mouth of the strong odors of food and bad breath.

To the Chinese, fruits are said to balance the "yin and yang" of the body. They believe that yin (cold energy) and yang (warm energy) should be balanced to maintain a healthy body.

Yang (warm energy) foods generally contain plenty of protein and fat such as meat, eggs, cheese and seafood. The method of cooking such as baking and deep-frying are said to increase yang.

Yin (cold energy) foods are mainly those that contain more water such as fruits and vegetables. Steaming and boiling food increase yin.

Food with a balanced yin and yang energy is said to be neutral in energy. Examples of such food are grains and beans.

Chinese mothers will insist that their children, who usually like deep-fried food, must eat fruit at the end of the meal. They believe too much fried or yang food will cause sore throats, cold blisters and an overall weak immune system.

The Chinese have believed this for many centuries before western scientists found that fruits are indeed rich in essential vitamins and minerals.

The Chinese also believe it is important to have a bowel movement at least once every day. One of the first questions a Chinese doctor (herbalist) will ask a patient is if the patient has a regular bowel movement. If it is not regular, the doctor will prescribe some herbs with a cooling effect and suggest that the patient eat a lot of fruit to clean the body and the digestive system.

Now scientists know that fruit can help bowel movements because it is rich in fiber. And since fiber cannot break down in our stomachs, we get a discount in calories when we eat high-fiber food.

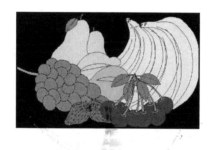

Fruits are high in fiber

Eating fruit in its natural form is more beneficial for weight loss than drinking fruit juices or eating fruit sauces. A study by Obbagy and Rolls in 2008 on the effect of fruit in different form on energy intake and satiety at a meal which involved 68 participants in a cross-over design with repeated measures found that subject consumed significantly less energy from the test meal after eating apple segments compared to the applesauce and apple juice preloads. They also consumed less energy after eating applesauce compared to after drinking apple juice.

Varieties of Asian Exotic Fruits

Enjoy fruit as your dessert and you will lose weight, have "sweet" breath, and reduce your risk of heart diseases, constipation and colon cancer.

Below are a few tropical fruits that are increasingly available in the local or Asian supermarkets:

Mango: ripe when the color is yellow or red and is slightly soft when you squeeze it. However, if it is too soft, it may be already rotten. Peel the skin and enjoy the flesh. Ripe mango tastes sweet while unripe mango tastes sour. You can still enjoy the sour mango if you add caramel and peanut butter sauce. See the recipe in Chapter 12.

Papaya: just like mango, ripe papaya is yellowish or reddish and is slightly soft. First cut them in half, throw away the seeds, then peel the skin and cut the meat into bite-size pieces.

Guava: ripe when the flesh is slightly soft. The skin is edible. Some believe the seeds might cause appendicitis and avoid them. I eat every part of it and at age 37, I have not had appendicitis, so it is your call!

Lychee: you can find this fruit fresh or canned in an Asian market. Peel off the skin and enjoy the sweet white flesh. The seed is not edible.

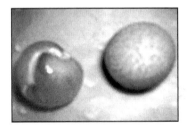

Longan: just like lychee, this fruit might be available fresh, frozen or canned in an Asian market. The skin and the seed are not edible. The meat has a transparent shade.

Jackfruit: some Vietnamese markets sell fresh jackfruit. However, it is a hassle to peel them since they are surrounded by a sticky outer layer. Most Asian markets sell peeled frozen or canned jackfruit. The flesh is yellow and the seed is not edible.

Star fruit (carambola): ripe when the edges are slightly brown. The skin is edible but not the seed.

Durian: you can only find this exotic fruit in large Asian markets. It is exotic because of the shape and smell. It has spikes all over it and the smell is so strong that airline operators in Asia banned it from the cabin area. The flesh is yellow, very rich and sweet. It is considered a delicacy. However, natives believe too much durian can make a person sick.

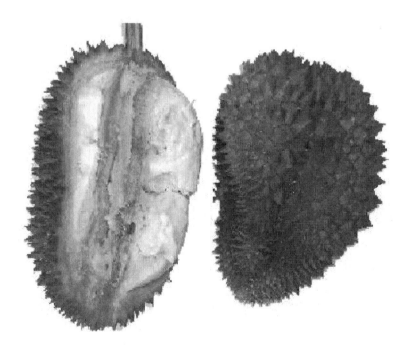

Durian

Tasty and Healthy Snacks Sold by Fast Food Vendors in Asia (Yes, we do have fast food, even more than in America!)

Other than cut-up fruits, the food vendors in Asia also sell a variety of other snacks such as:

Boiled or grilled corn
Corn on a cob is a popular snack in Asia. It is eaten plain or with a mixture of salt, chili and lime juice.
A friend of mine came up with this crispy boiled corn idea:
1. Heat corn in the microwave for 5 minutes.
2. Grill corn in the toaster oven for 3 minutes. Enjoy!

Boiled or broiled yams
Boiled or grilled yam is another popular snack. Eat it plain or with a mixture of salt and chili sauce.

Bananas
Asians love bananas. They are boiled, grilled, stewed with syrup or deep-fried.

In Asia, we cook burro, a kind of banana that looks like a short plantain. However, you can use regular bananas or plantains and get almost the same taste.

Boiled banana: boil a slightly unripe banana with skin in a pot with plenty of water for 2 minutes. Drain, and eat while the banana still warm. Alternatively, you can heat the banana for 1 minutes in the microwave.

Fried banana: coat a peeled banana with tempura flour and deep-fry it.

Grilled banana: put the peeled banana in a nonstick pan or toaster oven, spray with cooking oil and cook until the banana is slightly brown. Enjoy with maple or homemade brown sugar syrup.

Banana stewed with syrup: see the recipe in Chapter 12.

Beans, grains or fruits in sweet sauce
Green or red beans, black rice, barley, and starchy roots are cooked with white or brown sugar and water to create a sweet soup.

Mixed fruit with shaved or crushed ice
You will find this cold dessert to be as refreshing as ice cream at a fraction of the calories and fat.

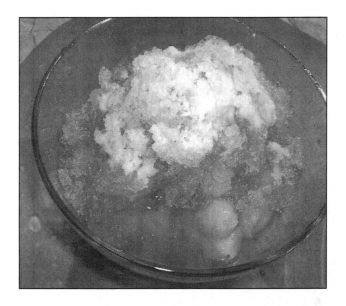

Mixed fruit with shaved ice and strawberry syrup.

If your children don't like fruits try to serve them this way. Wal-mart sells an ice shaving ice machine for about $25. Alternatively you can use a blender to make crushed ice.

Most Asian Snacks are Healthier than American Snacks

- **They are made of unprocessed food.**
  Example:

Unprocessed Food	Calories	Fat(g)	Fiber(g)
1 corn on the cob	80	1	2
1 medium apple	80	0	5
Processed Food			
1 oz. corn chips	160	10	1
1 cup apple sauce	200	0	2

Processed food is higher in calories and fat, and lower in fiber and water content.

When you eat natural, unprocessed food you will feel full with lesser calories for these reasons:

- **Unprocessed food contains more water.** Thus, it is larger in volume and will fill you up more quickly.

- **Unprocessed food contains more fiber.** Fiber is hard to digest and keeps the stomach full for a longer time thus delaying the return of hunger. The fiber eventually will be excreted from the body as waste.

- **Asian snacks are rich in complex carbohydrates (good carbs).** Complex carbohydrates have a complex structure. Our bodies have to work hard to digest complex carbohydrates (good carbs). Good carbs stay longer in our bodies, keeping us full and reducing our cravings for sugar.

- **Most snacks are made of plants and are rich in fiber and resistant starches.** Our bodies cannot absorb the calories from fiber and resistant starch. Furthermore, as discussed in Chapter 3, resistant starch increases fat oxidation and reduces the presence of fat in the body.

Some Asian snacks are as sinful as American snacks. Asians also enjoy cookies and cakes. However, they enjoy the sweets with hot tea or coffee.

Enjoy sweets with a hot drink and you will be satisfied with a smaller amount.

Hot drinks imitate the effect that soup has on the stomach. The stomach senses the presence of warm food and will immediately feel fuller.

Build Up Slimming Habits

- **Enjoy various fruits as your desserts or snacks.**
Fruits are high in fiber, low in calories and leave a feeling of "sweet breath" in your mouth.

- **Replace high-calorie snacks with unprocessed food.**
Eat boiled (or microwaved) corn, yams and grilled bananas. These warm snacks keep you full and satisfied with a lot less calories and fat.

- **Stock fresh, frozen and canned fruit at home.**
Canned fruit might contain heavy syrup so dilute or drain the syrup. The fruits do retain some of the vitamins and fiber.

Avoid dried fruits which are usually rich in calories because of the added sugar.

- **Clean out processed foods such as chips and candies from your pantry.** When you have the cravings just buy a small-sized portion. A bigger bag is never a good deal for your health. Remember, buying food in bulk is cheap but doctor bills and prescription drugs are not!

- **Adding fresh or canned fruit to your regular high-calorie dessert will make you feel satisfied with fewer calories.**
For example: add fruit cocktail to your ice cream or jello.

- **Get the low-calorie alternative to your favorite dessert.**
One day, out of curiosity, I compared the Ben and Jerry's regular ice cream in Cherry Garcia flavor with their frozen yogurt of the same flavor. To my surprise, they tasted exactly the same!

Yang = warm energy

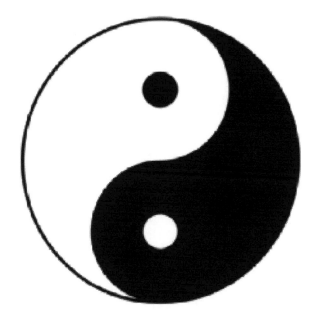

Yin = cold energy

Balance your food intake for optimum health.

10
Drinks to Keep You Slim

One of the biggest differences between the Asian and American diet is the beverages. Asians drink hot or iced unsweetened tea or water during meals and throughout the day while most Americans consume high-calorie drinks:

☹ Juice, 120 calories/glass

☹ Soda, 150 calories/can

☹ Coffee, 110–150 calories/cup

☹ Beer, 140 calories/can

☹ Wine, 90 calories/4 fl. oz. wine glass

Drinks Can Make You Fat More Quickly Than Foods. Why?

Your stomach has a limited capacity. When you are full, you cannot eat any more for some time because the food needs to be digested.

However, you have an unlimited ability to drink. Liquids, especially cold drinks, pass through the stomach quickly. They contribute calories from their sugar or alcohol content to the body and then go directly to the kidneys to be expelled. As long as you empty your kidneys, you have a virtually unlimited ability to consume calories through drinks.

Free resources: www.asianslimsecrets.com

Calculate the Calories from Drinks

If you drink a can of soda every day:
1 can of soda = 150 calories
150 calories x 365 days = 54,750 calories.

Since 1 pound = 3500 calories, 54,750 calories is equal to 16 pounds.

If you skip a can of soda every day, in a year you will reduce your calorie intake by the equivalent of 16 pounds!

If you skip a juice, coffee, beer, or wine every day you can easily reduce your calorie intake by the equivalent of 10–15 pounds a year even without changing your eating habits!

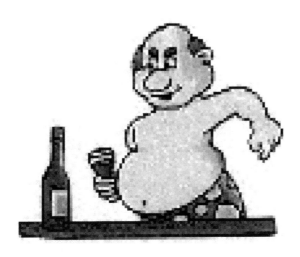

Guess... where does the beer belly come from?

Eat Your Fruit Instead of Drinking It

A glass of unsweetened orange juice is made from four oranges and it contains 120 calories. An orange contains only 30 calories. If you eat four oranges you will consume the same amount of calories but you will feel full for a longer time because of the fiber in the fruits.

When fruits are processed to become juice, they lose the fiber. Hence, juice does not fill you up.

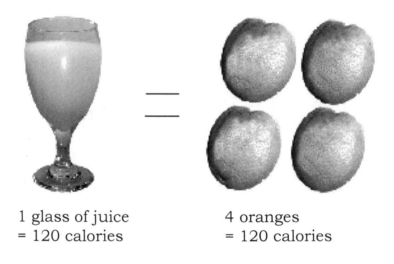

1 glass of juice
= 120 calories

4 oranges
= 120 calories

Juice, smoothies and milkshakes are high in calories.

Average calories per 16 fl. oz.

Apple juice	240
Smoothies (fruit only)	210
Smoothies (fruit+milk)	350
Milkshake	580

How about the Liquid Diet?

Many people try to lose weight by drinking juice or liquid meal replacement products. Scientific studies show that liquid diet is not an effective method to lose weight.

Mattes and Campbell (2009) study the effects of food form and timing of ingestion on appetite and energy intake in adults. In the cross over study, the partici pants consume 300 kcal of a solid food (apple), semi solid (apple sauce) and beverage (apple juice) at a meal or 2 hours later as a snack. The result shows that whether consumed with a meal or alone as a snack, the beverage elicited the weakest appetitive response, the solid food form elicited the strongest appetitive response and the semisolid response was intermediate.

Stull et al. (2008) compared how liquid and solid meal replacement products affect appetite and food intake in older adults in a within subject design study. They gave subjects either a liquid meal replacement product or a solid meal replacement product and after 2 hours served subjects with a test meal. They found that sub jects consumed more calories after the liquid meal replace-ment product than the solid meal replacement product.

Tea

Asians drink hot tea with their meal or snack. They believe hot tea helps to digest fatty food.

Hot plain tea contains 0 calories and has many benefits. It is also filling. A cup of hot tea in the afternoon might help you avoid or reduce fatty snacks.

Current research shows that tea offers a lot of health benefits:

- **Fights Cancer**
  Tea is rich in antioxidants that help the body to fight cancer. Many studies have shown that tea consumption reduce the development of skin cancer (Hakim and Harris, 2001), prostate cancer (Jatoi, Ellison, Burch et al, 2003 and Jian, Xie, Lee, Binns, 2004), lung cancer (Hakim, Harris, Brown et al. , 2003), breast cancer (Sun, Yuan, Koh and Yu, 2006) , colon and liver cancer (Sueoka,Suganuma, Sueoka, 2001 and Su, Arab, 2002)

- **Prevent Arthritis**
  A study in Britain found that older women who drank tea had significantly greater (approximately 5%) bone mineral density than those who did not drink tea (Hegarty, May and Khaw, 2000).

- **Lower the Risk of Heart Disease**
  In a meta-analysis of 9 studies involving 194,965 people and 4378 strokes, the data showed that individuals who consumed more than or equal to 3 cups of tea/day had a 21% lower risk of stroke than those who consumed less than 1 cup/day, regardless of their country of origin (Arab, Liu and Elashoff, 2009).

- **Makes You Look Younger**
  Antioxidants also help slow down the aging process.

- **Fights Germs and Boosts Immune System**
  Tea is rich in alkylamines which are germ-fighting chemicals.

- **Improves Digestion**
  Tea increases the flow of digestive juices to help the digestion of fatty food.

- **Prevents Food Poisoning**
  Catachins found in tea prevent food poisoning by killing germs and bacteria in the stomach.

- **Protects Teeth & Strengthens Bones**
  Tea contains fluoride to protect teeth and strengthen bones.

- **Rich in several minerals that are vital for the body** such as potassium, manganese and zinc

What if I Don't Like Water or Tea?

- Try some flavored herbal tea. Add some ice or even 1 tablespoon of sugar, 48 calories, which is still less calories than your regular soda.

- Enjoy your meal with 2 glasses of liquid, one water and one sugary drink. When you are very thirsty and need a big gulp, drink the water. Savor the sugary drink a little at a time, like when you sip wine.

- Dilute your favorite drink with some water or get flavored water which has zero calories.

- Learn to live with diet drinks. Soda companies keep improving the taste of their diet products. Also, after a while, most people get used to the diet alternative.

Build Up Slimming Habits

- Choose your drink as carefully as when you select your food. Drinks can make you fat faster than food.

- Drink zero or low-calorie liquid: water, flavored water, hot tea, unsweetened cold tea, diet soda.

- Hot drinks make you full. Drinking a cup of hot tea or hot water before you eat might help you control your cravings.

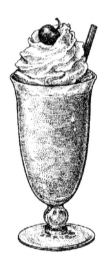

Drinks can make you fat!
16 fl. oz. milkshake contains
580 calories, 17 g fat.

Free resources: www.asianslimsecrets.com

11
Turn Back the Clock and Increase Your Metabolism

Most Asians who eat their food the traditional way as described in the previous chapters are slim. However, as they age and reach their sixties, some begin to gain extra weight. Even though an obese Asian is a rare sight, older Asians typically gain 10–30 pounds in their retirement years.

In Asia, senior centers are rare. Classes or activities directed at older adults are few. In heavily populated countries such as Singapore, Hong Kong and Japan, houses are small and there is no backyard for gardening or room for a pet. Many seniors pass their time sitting around, chatting with the neighbors and watching TV.

As a result, these seniors lose lean muscle. Since lean muscle is the calorie-eating machine of your body, losing it will create a surplus of calories. This surplus is deposited as fat tissue. Pound per pound, lean muscle tissue consumes 50 more calories than fat tissue in a day. If you lose 2 pounds of lean muscle tissue, you lose the capacity to burn an extra 100 calories in a day or 36,500 calories in a year. Since 1 pound is equal to 3,500 calories, losing that 2 pounds of muscle could make you gain about 10 pounds of fat a year.

This is why it is easier for older people to gain weight. In fact, after our 25th birthday, we start to lose about 10% of our lean muscle every year. So, when we are older and still eat the same amount of calories as when we were 25 years of age, we will gain weight because our body doesn't need as many calories.

The best way to reverse the clock is to increase your muscle. When you gain muscle, your body will burn more calories and lose weight.

To efficiently increase muscle, strength training is promoted in many books and gyms nowadays for several reasons:

1. More muscle means more calories are consumed 24 hours a day, 7 days a week. Muscular people burn more calories than nonmuscular ones even when they are sleeping or watching TV.

Sleeping for 8 hours

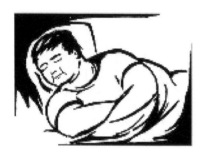   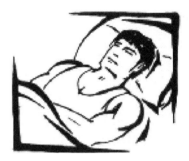

Less muscle   More muscle
burns 400 calories   burns 600 calories

2. Strength training has a low injury risk. Running, walking and high impact aerobics can put too much stress on your foot joints, especially if you are already overweight. They are also not efficient. To lose 1 pound, you need to walk 35 miles or an hour every day for seven days a week. If you prefer to walk, increase your muscles and metabolism by carrying small weights.

3. Strength training is more time efficient and can be done indoors. In the next few pages you will learn movements you can do while watching TV, waiting in line, or brushing your teeth.

4. Strength training strengthens your bones.

5. Strength training, as long as it is not done excessively, will not make you look like Arnold Schwarzenegger. You will look firm and toned, but not bulky.

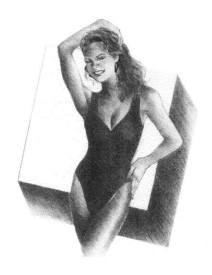

Firm, but not bulky

Important Notes About Strength Training

1. Warm up
To reduce the risk of injury, you need to warm up your muscles. Move the muscles you are going to use. Walk in place, lifting your knee and swinging your arms high for a couple of minutes.

2. Proper position
Pay special attention to the correct position. A wrong position, such as over-arching your back, can lead to injury.

3. Remember to breathe
Remember to inhale and exhale as you do the movements. Holding your breath may cause your blood pressure to shoot up and could be fatal for people who have a heart condition.

4. Lift and lower slowly
To work out the muscle correctly, lift and lower the weight slowly. In fact, the slower the movement, the harder your muscles have to work against gravity.

5. Rest period
Do not work on the same muscle two days in a row. After training, give the particular muscle at least 24 hours rest. During the rest period, the muscle will repair itself and grow stronger.

Calves

You can strengthen your calves while brushing your teeth.

1. Raise your heels and stand on your toes.
2. Hold for 30–60 seconds while breathing normally.
3. Lower your heels down slowly. Repeat a few times.

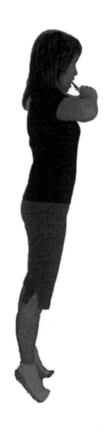

Buttocks

You can tone your buttocks while waiting in front of the microwave.

1. Stand up straight. Squeeze your buttock muscles tightly for 10 seconds. Breath normally.
2. Relax and repeat 10–20 times.

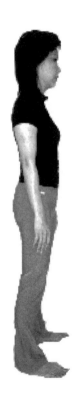 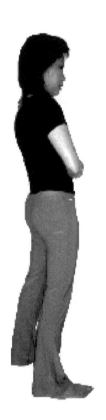

Quadriceps

Telephone time is perfect for working out your quadriceps.

1. Stand against a wall.
2. Slowly move your feet forward and let your back slide down the wall as if you are about to sit in a chair. Your knees should not stick out past your feet, but should form a right angle.
3. Hold this position for 10–20 seconds, then go back to your original position.
4. Rest for 10 seconds and repeat the movement as long as you are still on the phone. When your feet and quadriceps are killing you, maybe it's time to stop talking!

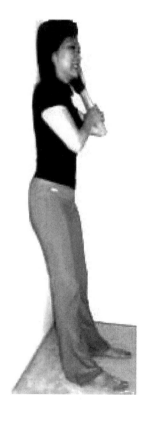 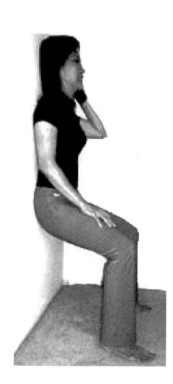

Abs

This is something you can do discreetly while waiting in the doctor's office or standing in line.

1. Stand or sit up straight.
2. Pull in and tighten your stomach for 5 seconds while continue to breathe normally. Release and repeat 20–30 times.

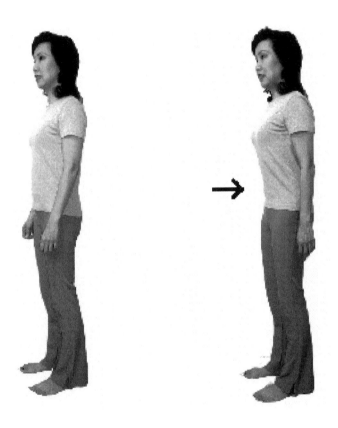

Outer Thigh

In bed at night, it's not too late to do a little exercise.

1. Lie on your side.
2. Lift and lower one leg slowly. Do 10 repetitions (1 set).
3. Rest, alternate legs. Do 2–3 sets.

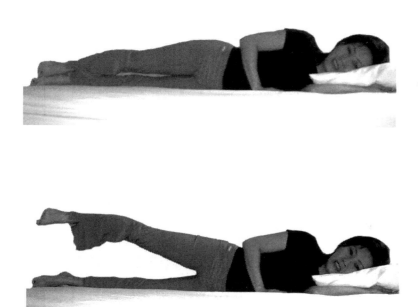

Upper Thigh

1. Lie on your back.
2. Bend one knee and keep one foot on the floor.
3. Lift and lower the other leg slowly. Do 10 repetitions (1 set).
4. Rest and alternate legs. Do 2–3 sets.

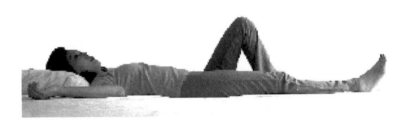

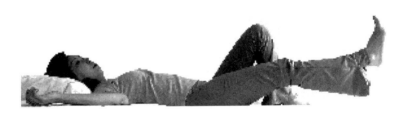

Dumbbells

For the following exercises you will need a dumbbell. Alternatively you may use a bottle of water but since dumbbells are inexpensive ($2–$5) and they are easier to grab, they are good investments.

How to Select the Perfect Weight

It's very important to select the right weight because if the weight is too light, it will not work out your muscles. If it's too heavy, you might injure them.

Do the bicep curl as shown below:
1. Hold a dumbbell with palm facing forward.
2. Lift and lower it down slowly.

The perfect weight is the one that makes your muscle feel fatigued after you curl 12 times continuously.

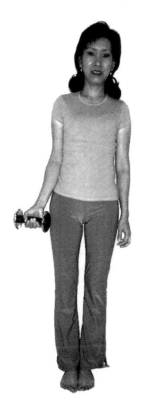 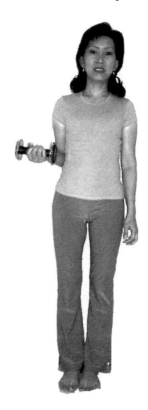

Hammer Curl

These are my favorite movements since I can do them while watching TV.

1. Hold the dumbbell steadily; do not let it wiggle.
2. Lift and lower it down slowly.
3. Do 10 repetitions (1 set). Alternate with the other arm. Do 2–3 sets.

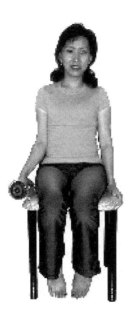 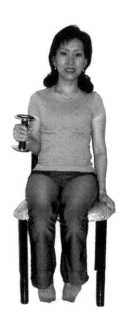

Triceps Curl

1. With both hands, hold the bar of the dumbbell with the palms up.
2. Slowly raise the dumbbell above your head and lower to the starting position. Do 10 repetitions (1 set).
3. Repeat 2–3 sets with one minute rest between sets.

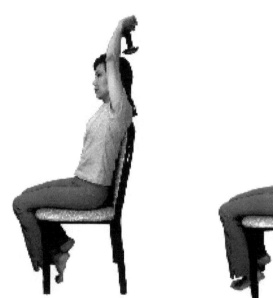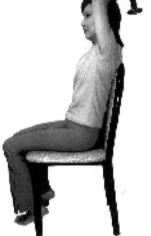

Shoulder

1. Grab a dumbbell in each hand firmly. Do not wiggle.
2. Sit straight; do not slouch.
3. Bend your elbows and with your dumbbells at ear level, slowly lift them.
4. Keep your elbows relaxed, do not lock your joints. Slowly lower the dumbbell to starting position.
5. Repeat 10 times (1 set). Do 2–3 sets with rest between sets.

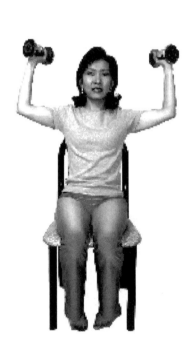 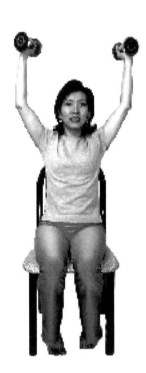

Free resources: www.asianslimsecrets.com

Back Muscles

1. Grab a dumbbell in each hand.
2. Sit on a chair with your chest slightly leaning forward.
3. With your wrists stable and using strength from your shoulder and upper back muscles, pull both dumbbells up with your elbows pointing backward as high as you can.
4. Slowly lower the dumbbell while breathing normally.
5. Repeat 10 times (1 set). Rest for a minute and do 2–3 sets.

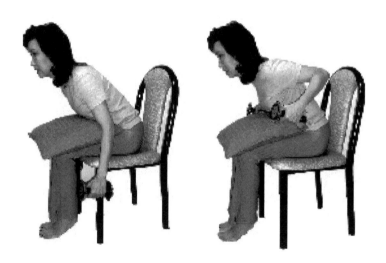

Build Up Slimming Habits

- Buy a pair of dumbbells.

- Do simple exercises while watching TV, brushing your teeth, talking on the phone, etc.

- **Commit to at least 10 minutes of strength training as part of your daily rituals.** If you have time to brush your teeth twice a day to maintain healthy teeth, realize that maintaining your entire body is even more beneficial.

When health is absent

Wisdom cannot reveal itself,

Art cannot become manifest,

Strength cannot be exerted,

Wealth is useless, and

Reason is powerless.

Herophilies, 300 B.C.

12

Favorite Recipes from Thailand, Hong Kong, Singapore, Japan, Korea, Indonesia and Vietnam

I spent some time observing the eating habits of Asians and non-Asians in the workplace. Asians usually eat big meals that include rice or noodles with meat or fish and vegetables. Their staple food is the same but the items served with their rice or noodles changes daily. Non-Asians tend to have a more predictable menu, and some even eat the same thing every day: turkey, ham or peanut butter sandwiches, or maybe salad or fruit with cottage cheese.

After lunch, the Asians are satisfied with their meal and pass by the vending machine without any interest while their non-Asian coworkers are easily tempted by the various high-fat, high-calorie snacks.

Enjoy great food and a variety of dishes at mealtime to keep you full and satisfied so you won't be easily tempted to grab fattening snacks.

Try the following recipes to bring more "spice" to your plate.

I. Rice and Noodles

II. Soup

III. Meat, Seafood, Tofu and Egg

IV. Vegetables

V. Snacks and Dessert

I. Rice and Noodles

Steamed White Rice

Servings: 6
Steamed white rice is a staple food in Asia. No meal is complete without it. Leftovers can be reheated in the microwave or used as an ingredient for fried rice.

2 cups long/short grain white rice, washed and
  drained
3 cups water
If you like softer rice (like sushi) use 4 cups of water

Heat rice and water in a pot until the water boils.

Stir rice gently, turn to medium-low heat and cover the pot. Simmer for 15 minutes or longer until all of the water has been absorbed and rice is cooked.

Note: Don't stir the rice while cooking at low heat because stirring will make it stick together. Covering the pot while cooking at low heat is important to maintain a perfect balance of heat and steam pressure inside the pot.

Per serving: 225 calories, 0 fat (0 g saturated fat),
4 g protein, 49 g carbohydrates, 1 g dietary fiber.

Free resources: www.asianslimsecrets.com

Steamed Brown Rice

Servings: 6
Brown rice contains more vitamins than white rice. To improve the taste, add some chicken broth (bouillon).

2 cups brown rice, washed and drained
4 cups water
2 tablespoons chicken broth powder, optional

Heat rice, chicken broth and water in a pot until the water boils.

Stir rice gently, turn to medium-low heat and cover the pot. Simmer for 40 minutes or longer until all of the water has been absorbed and rice is cooked.

Note: As with the white rice, don't stir the rice while cooking at low heat, and keep pot covered to maintain the balance of heat and steam pressure.

Per serving: 235 calories, 2 g fat (0 g saturated fat), 5 g protein, 49 g carbohydrates, 1 g dietary fiber.

Fried Rice

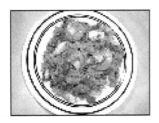

Servings: 4
Fried rice is a meal by itself. It is also a great way to use the leftover steamed rice.

6 ounces skinless boneless chicken breast or peeled shrimp.
4 tablespoons soy sauce
2 whole eggs, lightly beaten
3 tablespoons vegetable oil
4 tablespoons chopped green onions or onion
4 cups cooked rice
1 cup frozen peas and carrots
salt and pepper to taste

If using chicken, cut into thinly sliced pieces. Marinade with 1 tbsp. soy sauce for 10 minutes.

Put ½ tsp. oil and the 2 eggs in the pan to make scrambled eggs. Sprinkle with salt and pepper and set aside.

Again, drop ½ tsp. oil in the pan to stir fry the chicken or shrimp until cooked. Set aside.

Heat the remaining oil in the pan, stir fry green onions for 1 minute, add rice and 3 tbsp. soy sauce; mix well.

Add peas and carrots, chicken or shrimp and egg. Continue to mix for a few minutes. Add salt and pepper to taste. Serve.

Per serving: 440 calories, 14 g fat (2 g saturated fat), 20 g protein, 58 g carbohydrates, 2 g dietary fiber.

California Sushi Rolls

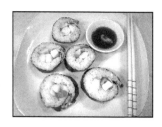

Servings : 5
This sushi roll originate in California. It combines rice, imitation crab, cucumber and avocado.

2 cups short grain rice, washed and drained
4 cups water
2 tablespoons dry white wine or sake
3 tablespoons rice wine vinegar or white vinegar
3 tablespoons sugar
½ teaspoon salt
1 ounce nori or dried seaweed
½ pound imitation crab stick
4 ounces avocado, peeled and cut in thin strips
½ medium cucumber, peeled and cut in thin strips
5 tablespoons soy sauce
1 teaspoon wasabi, optional

Boil rice, water and wine in a pot. Stir, then cover the pot tightly. Simmer on medium-low heat for 20 minutes. Transfer the cooked rice to a big bowl.

Put vinegar, sugar and salt in a small bowl and mix well. Pour over rice and mix again. Fan rice to cool down.

Cut a piece of plastic wrap about the size of 12 x 12 inches. Put a sheet of dried seaweed on top of the plastic.

Spread sushi rice on top of the seaweed. Place a piece of crab stick, cucumber strip and avocado strip on top of the rice

Roll the sushi tightly and use the plastic to make sausage-like shape. Cut the roll into ¾-inch pieces, then remove plastic wrap. Serve sushi with soy sauce and wasabi paste.

Per serving: 418 calories, 4 g fat (1 g saturated fat), 12 g protein, 80 g carbohydrates, 3 g dietary fiber.

Rice Porridge (Congee)

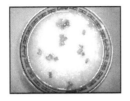

Servings: 4
Rice porridge is commonly eaten as breakfast or a snack.

5 cups water
2 tablespoons chicken broth powder
1½ cup white grain rice, rinsed and drained
½ pound lean pork/chicken/fish, sliced to thin pieces
1 teaspoon cornstarch
½ teaspoon sugar
2 tablespoons soy sauce
2 tablespoons minced spring onions, optional

You can reduce cooking time by using steamed rice instead. Mix 3 cups rice and 1 cup water in a blender. With this method, the cooking time of porridge is reduced to 15 minutes.

Heat water, chicken broth and rice until it boils. Reduce the heat to medium and cook with the lid on for 35 minutes. Stir the mixture occasionally so the rice does not stick to the pot.

In a bowl, marinate meat with cornstarch, sugar and soy sauce. Set aside.

When the porridge is cooked, add the meat and boil for 5–10 minutes. Serve warm and garnish with spring onions.

Per serving: 340 calories, 3 g fat (1 g saturated fat), 18 g protein, 58 g carbohydrates, 1 g dietary fiber.

Thai Fried Noodles (Shrimp Pad Thai)

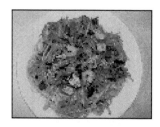

Servings: 4
A popular Thai noodle dish with shrimp and egg, sprinkled with chopped roasted peanuts.

½ pound rice noodles or pasta of your choice
4 teaspoons vegetable oil
4 ounces shrimps, peeled
2 large eggs, lightly beaten
3 tablespoon fish sauce
1 tablespoon sugar
½ teaspoon salt
1 tablespoon chili sauce or chili powder, optional
2 tablespoons soy sauce
1 tablespoon minced garlic
2 stalks green onions, chopped
4 ounces bean sprouts
4 tablespoons peanuts, coarsely chopped
1 teaspoon lime juice or vinegar

Cook noodles as instructed by the package. Then rinse with cold water to prevent overcooking and drain.

Heat ½ tsp. oil in the pan, cook shrimp for 2 minutes or until pink, and set aside. Skip this step if you use cooked shrimp.

Heat ½ tsp. oil and add eggs to make scrambled eggs. Sprinkle salt to taste and set aside.

In a bowl, combine fish sauce, sugar, salt, chili and soy sauces.

Heat 3 tsp. vegetable oil in the pan. Stir-fry garlic and green onions for 30 seconds. Add noodles, bean sprouts and the sauce mixture; toss to mix. Add eggs, shrimps, peanuts and lime juice. Serve.

Per serving: 456 calories, 17 g fat (3 g saturated fat), 14 g protein, 62 g carbohydrates, 2 g dietary fiber.

Yellow Rice

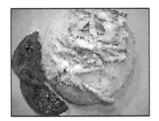

Servings: 6
This fragrant rice goes well with a scrambled egg.

2 cups white rice, washed and drained
2 teaspoons vegetable oil
2 teaspoons minced onion
2 teaspoons minced garlic
3 cups water
½ teaspoon turmeric powder
2 teaspoon salt
4 tablespoons coconut oil

Heat oil in a pot, stir-fry onion and garlic for 1 minute. Add rice, water, turmeric, salt and coconut oil.

Bring to a boil. Stir gently and reduce to medium-low heat.

Cover the pot tightly and simmer for 20 minutes.

Per serving: 264 calories, 4 g fat (2 g saturated fat), 5 g protein, 50 g carbohydrates, 1 g dietary fiber.

Beef Fried Noodles (Lo Mein)

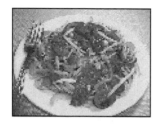

Servings: 4
*Quick stir-fry noodles with beef
and vegetables.*

½ pound noodles or pasta, cooked and drained
½ pound lean beef, sliced thin
4 tablespoons soy sauce
2 tablespoons dry sherry or rice wine
1 teaspoon sesame oil
½ teaspoon salt
1½ tablespoon vegetable oil
2 stalks green onions, chopped
1 tablespoon minced garlic
4 ounces mushroom sliced
1 stalk celery, chopped
4 ounces bean spouts

Marinate beef with 2 tbsp. soy sauce for 15 minutes.

In a small bowl, combine sherry, 2 tbsp. soy sauce, salt
and sesame oil. Set aside.

Heat the pan with ½ tbsp. oil to stir-fry beef until it is
cooked. Transfer it to a plate.

Heat 1 tbsp. oil in the pan to stir fry green onions, garlic,
mushrooms, celery and bean sprouts for 2 minutes. Stir
in the soy sauce mixture, add cooked beef and noodles.
Continue to stir-fry for 1 minute. Serve.

Per serving: 433 calories, 17 g fat (4 g saturated fat),
22 g protein, 47 g carbohydrates, 3 g fiber.

Chicken Noodles Indonesian Style (Mie Ayam)

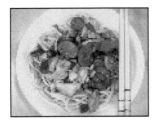

Servings: 4
Noodles with chicken, mush-
room and oyster sauce.

12 ounces instant noodles or pasta of your choice,
   cooked and drained
1 tablespoon fish sauce or 1½ teaspoon soy sauce
½ tablespoon vegetable oil
1 tablespoon minced garlic
½ pound skinless boneless chicken breast, cut in
   ½-inch cubes
3 tablespoons oyster sauce
1 cup straw mushrooms or regular sliced mushrooms
2 tablespoons chopped green onions to garnish,
   optional

Cook and drain noodles as instructed. Pour fish sauce
on the noodles and mix well. Arrange noodles on individual serving plates.

Heat oil in a pan to stir-fry garlic, chicken breast and
oyster sauce for 5 minutes or until the chicken is
cooked.

Add mushrooms and continue to stir-fry for a couple
of minutes. Pour the mixture on top of the noodles and
serve.

Per serving: 422 calories, 7 g fat (1 g saturated fat),
26 g protein, 64 g carbohydrates, 2 g dietary fiber.

Japanese Noodle Soup (Udon)

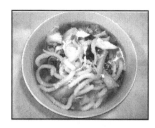

Servings: 4
Noodles and vegetables in clear chicken broth.

12 ounces Japanese udon noodles or pasta of your choice
6 ounces skinless boneless chicken breast or imitation crabmeat, sliced thin
1 teaspoon vegetable oil
1 tablespoon minced ginger
1 tablespoon minced garlic
2 tablespoons soy sauce
4 cups water
2 tablespoons chicken broth powder
4 ounces mushrooms or shitake mushrooms, sliced thin
1 cup bok choy or green leafy vegetable of your choice, chopped
2 stalks green onions, chopped
2 tablespoon sake or white wine

Prepare noodles as directed by the package. Drain and set aside.

Heat oil in the pan, stir-fry ginger and garlic for 30 seconds. Add chicken and soy sauce, and stir-fry for 2 minutes.

Add water, chicken broth, mushrooms, bok choy, and green onions; simmer for 5 minutes. Stir in the noodles and sake. Serve.

Per serving: 418 calories, 6 g fat (1 g saturated fat), 24 g protein, 66 g carbohydrates, 3 g dietary fiber.

Vietnamese Beef Noodle Soup

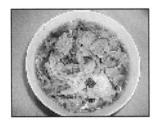

Servings: 4
Noodles and sliced beef in beef broth.

½ pound lean beef, slice very thin
8 ounces Vietnamese rice noodles or pasta of your
  choice
1 teaspoon vegetable oil
1 small onion, sliced thin
1 teaspoon grated ginger root
2 tablespoons beef broth powder
6 cups water
3 star anise or 2-inch cinnamon stick
1 teaspoon salt
1 teaspoon sugar
½ pound bean sprouts
Garnish (optional): lime wedges, chili sauce

Prepare rice noodles as directed by the package. Drain and rinse to prevent it from overcooking. Set aside.

Heat oil in the pot, stir-fry onion and ginger until fragrant. Add beef broth, water, star anise, salt and sugar. Simmer on medium heat for 15 minutes. Take out the star anise.

Add beef slices, and cook for 3 minutes. Add noodles and bean sprouts, then serve.

Per serving: 381 calories, 10 g fat (3 g saturated fat), 15 g protein, 58 g carbohydrates, 3 g dietary fiber.

II. Soup

Sweetcorn Soup

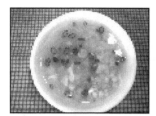

Servings: 4
Creamy corn soup thickened
with cornstarch and egg white.

2 tablespoons chicken broth powder
6 cups water
11 ounces canned or frozen corn
3 tablespoons cornstarch, mixed with ½ cup of water
1 egg white, beaten slightly
salt and pepper to taste
2 tablespoons chopped spring onions, to garnish

Boil water and chicken broth powder. Add corn and cornstarch solution. Stir gently for 3 minutes.

Add egg while continuing to stir the soup.

Bring soup to a boil again; add salt and pepper to taste. Garnish with spring onions and turn off the heat.

Per serving: 93 calories, 1 g fat (0 g saturated fat), 4 g protein, 20 g carbohydrates, 1 g dietary fiber.

Crabmeat and Asparagus Soup

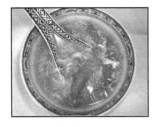

Servings: 4
Crabmeat and soft asparagus spears in a creamy egg flower soup

4 cups water
4 ounces crabmeat
12 ounces canned asparagus, cut in 2-inch slices
2 tablespoons cornstarch, dissolve in ½ cup water
1 egg, beaten
2 tablespoons oyster sauce or soy sauce
1 teaspoon salt
pepper to taste

Boil water and crabmeat in a pot.

Add asparagus and cornstarch solution. Stir gently while adding egg to form "the flower" in the soup.

Add oyster sauce, salt and pepper and cook until it boils. Serve.

Per serving: 74 calories, 2 g fat (0 g saturated fat), 9 g protein, 6 g carbohydrates, 1 g dietary fiber.

Chicken in Tumeric Soup (Soto Ayam)

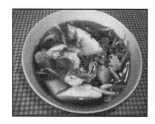

Servings: 4
Fragrant and filling chicken soup with the aroma of ginger, turmeric and coriander.

½ pound skinless boneless chicken breast, sliced thin
1 tablespoon minced garlic
2 tablespoons minced onion
1 tablespoon minced ginger
1 tablespoon vegetable oil
4 cups water
1 potato, peeled and cut into bite-size pieces
½ teaspoon turmeric powder
½ teaspoon coriander powder
2 teaspoon salt
¼ teaspoon pepper
5 ounces bean sprouts or sliced cabbage
1 teaspoon lime juice or vinegar
1 egg, hard-boiled and sliced

Marinate chicken slices with ½ teaspoon of salt and set aside.

Heat oil in a large pot to stir-fry garlic, onion and ginger for a minute. Add chicken, water, potato, tumeric, coriander, salt and pepper. Simmer for 15 minutes.

Add bean sprouts and lime juice; cook for 30 seconds. Garnish soup with egg slices.

Per serving: 151 calories, 5 g fat (1 g saturated fat), 16 g protein, 9 g carbohydrates, 1 g dietary fiber.

Thai Chicken and Coconut Milk Soup

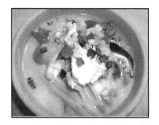

Servings: 4
An aromatic soup flavored with coconut milk, fish sauce and lemon juice.

½ pound skinless boneless chicken breast, sliced thin
1 teaspoon salt
½ teaspoon vegetable oil spray
1 teaspoon minced garlic
1 teaspoon grated ginger or galangal
4 cups water
2 tablespoons chicken broth powder
5 leaves kaffir lime leaves, cut in halves, optional
1 cup sliced mushrooms or straw mushrooms
1 cup canned bamboo shoots, sliced thin
1 cup corn
½ cup coconut milk
2 tablespoons lemon juice
2 tablespoon fish sauce
4 tablespoon chopped green onions, optional

Sprinkle salt on the chicken pieces.

Heat oil spray in the pot to stir-fry ginger, garlic and chicken for 2 minutes. Add water, chicken broth powder, kaffir lime leaves and simmer for 5 minutes.

Add mushrooms, bamboo shoots, corn and coconut milk. Simmer for 2 minutes, then add lemon juice and fish sauce.

Garnish with green onions and serve.

Per serving: 220 calories, 11 g fat (7 g saturated fat), 17 g protein, 17 g carbohydrates, 3 g dietary fiber.

Free resources: www.asianslimsecrets.com

Red Bean and Beef Soup

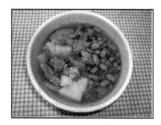

Servings : 4
Red beans, beef, potato and carrot in beef broth.

½ teaspoon vegetable oil spray
1 teaspoon minced garlic
6 ounces lean beef or pork, sliced thin
1 can cooked red kidney beans, drained
4 cups water
1 whole carrot, sliced
1 medium potato, cut in ½-inch cubes
½ teaspoon ground nutmeg
2 tablespoons beef broth powder
pepper to taste
4 tablespoons chopped green onions, to garnish

Heat vegetable oil in the pot, stir-fry garlic for 30 seconds. Add beef and continue to stir-fry for 1 minute.

Add water and the remaining of all the ingredients. Cook for 15 minutes, garnish with green onions and serve.

Per serving: 194 calories, 7 g fat (3 g saturated fat), 13 g protein, 19 g carbohydrates, 5 g dietary fiber.

Squash Soup

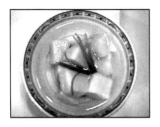

Servings: 4
This simple soup is great as an appetizer or a snack.

4 cups water
2 tablespoons chicken broth powder
1 tablespoon grated ginger root
1 pound butternut squash or other squash, peeled and
   cut into 1-inch cubes
salt and pepper to taste
1 tablespoon chopped green onions to garnish

Boil water, chicken broth powder, ginger and squash for about 15 minutes or until the squash becomes soft.

Add salt and pepper to taste and garnish with green onions if you like. Serve.

Per serving: 46 calories, 0 g fat (0 g saturated fat), 1 g protein, 12 g carbohydrates, 2 g dietary fiber.

Miso Soup

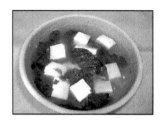

Servings: 4
This is a popular Japanese bean paste soup. Some local supermarkets carry the instant miso seasoning.

4 cups water
2 tablespoons fish stock or soy sauce
4 tablespoons miso
12 ounces tofu, cut in ½-inch cubes
2 cups spinach, cut 2 inches long

Bring water, fish stock and miso to a boil.

Add tofu and spinach, bring to a boil again, then turn off the heat.

Per serving: 107 calories, 5 g fat (1 g saturated fat), 9 g protein, 7 g carbohydrates, 2 g dietary fiber.

III. Meat, Seafood, Tofu and Egg Dishes

Chicken in Red Curry Sauce

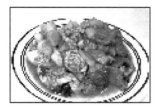

Servings: 4
Chicken and potato in a spicy curry sauce.

2 medium potatoes, peeled and cut into ½-inch cubes
1 tablespoon vegetable oil
1½ tablespoons red curry paste
12 ounces boneless skinless chicken breast/lean beef/
  seafood of your choice, sliced thin
¼ cup water
2 carrots, peeled and sliced thin
2 tablespoons fish sauce
2 tablespoons brown sugar
1 tablespoon lime juice
½ cup basil leaves
½ teaspoon salt

Boil potato cubes for 10 minutes or until they are soft, then drain and set aside.

Heat oil in the pot, add curry paste and stir-fry for 1 minute. Add chicken, continue to stir-fry for 2 minutes.

Add water, carrots, potato cubes, fish sauce, brown sugar, salt, lime juice and basil leaves. Simmer for 3 minutes and serve.

Per serving: 243 calories, 9 g fat (1 g saturated fat), 22 g protein, 19 g carbohydrates, 2 g dietary fiber.

Beef with Broccoli

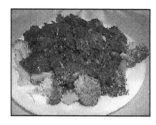

Servings: 4
Beef and broccoli in fragrant
oyster sauce with wine.

12 ounces lean beef, trimmed of all the visible fat and
   sliced thinly.
1 lb broccoli florets, cut into bite-size pieces
3 tablespoons oyster sauce
3 tablespoons soy sauce
1 tablespoon dry sherry or cooking wine
2 teaspoons minced garlic
2 tablespoons cornstarch
1 tablespoon vegetable oil
½ cup water
⅛ teaspoon salt

In a bowl, marinate beef with 2 tbsp. soy sauce, 1 tbsp.
oyster sauce, and 1 tbsp. cornstarch for about 10 minutes

In another bowl combine water, 1 tbsp. cornstarch, 1
tbsp. soy sauce, 2 tbsp. oyster sauce, salt and sherry.

Boil some water in a pot to cook broccoli for 2 minutes until crisp tender. Drain and transfer to a serving
plate.

Heat 1 tbsp. oil in a pan, stir-fry garlic for 30 seconds,
add beef and continue to stir-fry for 5 minutes. Add the
oyster sauce mixture and simmer until the sauce thickens. Pour beef mixture on top of broccoli and serve.

Per serving: 275 calories, 16 g fat (5 g saturated fat),
21 g protein, 12 g carbohydrates, 4 g dietary fiber.

Skewered Meat (Sate)

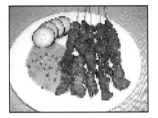

Servings: 4
Grilled skewered meat served with peanut sauce.

1 pound skinless boneless chicken breast or lean beef cut into 1-inch cubes
1 medium onion, minced
1 tablespoon grated ginger
1 tablespoon minced garlic
2 teaspoons ground coriander
1 teaspoon ground cumin
1 tablespoon vegetable oil
6 tablespoons soy sauce
3 tablespoons sugar
½ teaspoon salt
1 tablespoon peanut butter
1 tablespoon lemon juice
12 wood skewers, soaked in water for 20 minutes

Mix onion, ginger, garlic, coriander and cumin in a bowl. Heat oil in a pan and stir-fry the mixture for 2 minutes.

Marinate meat with the stir-fried seasonings, soy sauce, sugar, salt, peanut butter and lemon juice for at least 20 minutes. Thread several pieces of meat onto each skewer.

Cook sate on a grill or in an oven. Brushed meat with the marinating sauce, then turn so both sides are evenly cooked. Serve with peanut sauce (see recipe on the next page).

Note: If you are short on time you can stir-fry the meat, the seasonings and an extra 1 tbsp. peanut butter in a pan, eliminating the need to marinate and to make a separate peanut sauce. However, it is not as festive as eating them from the skewers.

Per serving: 379 calories, 24 g fat (8 g saturated fat), 23 g protein, 17 g carbohydrates, 1 g dietary fiber.

Peanut Sauce

Servings: 6
This sauce is made from peanut butter and is used as a condiment to sate or as a salad dressing.

1 teaspoon oil
1 teaspoon minced onion
1 teaspoon minced garlic
¾ cup water
3 tablespoons peanut butter
½ teaspoon crushed red pepper or chili sauce, optional
½ teaspoon coriander
½ teaspoon salt

Heat oil in the pan to stir-fry onion and garlic for 2 minutes.

Add the remaining ingredients and simmer until they form a thick mixture and serve.

Per serving: 55 calories, 5 g fat (1 g saturated fat), 2 g protein, 2 g carbohydrates, 0 g dietary fiber.

Chicken Teriyaki

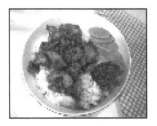

Servings: 4
Japanese-style grilled chicken
with sweet sauce.

12 ounces skinless boneless chicken breast, sliced thin
½ cup soy sauce
3 tablespoons sugar
1 teaspoon grated ginger
1 tablespoon sesame oil
1 teaspoon vegetable oil

Combine soy sauce, sugar and ginger in a bowl.

Heat oil in the pan or use cooking spray. Stir-fry the chicken while pouring the marinating sauce little by little to let the chicken absorb it slowly. Cook until the chicken is slightly brown and serve.

Per serving: 173 calories, 3 g fat (1 g saturated fat), 22 g protein, 13 g carbohydrates, 1 g dietary fiber.

Pork or Chicken Fillet with Lemon Grass

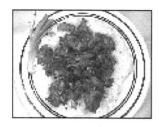

Servings: 4
Thai-style grilled meat with
subtle lemon flavor.

1 pound lean pork or chicken, sliced thin
1 stalk lemon grass, chopped fine, or 1 tablespoon
    grated lemon zest
2 stalks spring onions, chopped
3 tablespoons fish sauce
1 tablespoon vegetable oil
2 teaspoons minced garlic
1 teaspoon chili sauce or powder, optional
1 teaspoon sugar
1 teaspoon salt
¼ teaspoon pepper

Marinate meat with lemon grass, spring onions, 2 tbsp. fish sauce, salt and pepper for at least 15 minutes.

Heat oil in the pan. Stir-fry garlic and chili for 30 seconds. Add the meat and cook for 5 minutes.

Add sugar and 1 tbsp. fish sauce. Stir-fry until the meat is cooked and browned. Serve with steamed rice.

Per serving: 202 calories, 9 g fat (2 g saturated fat), 24 g protein, 5 g carbohydrates, 0 g dietary fiber.

Korean Grilled Meat

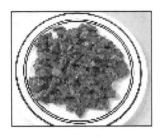

Servings: 4
Grilled meat with soy sauce,
sugar and sesame oil. Serve
with lettuce leaves and rice.

1 pound lean beef, sliced thin
3 tablespoons soy sauce
2 tablespoons sesame oil
2 tablespoons dry sherry or cooking wine
1 tablespoon sugar
¼ teaspoon pepper
1 medium onion, minced
1 tablespoon minced garlic
2 stalks green onions, chopped
½ teaspoon salt
2 ounces lettuce leaves

Mix the sliced beef with all the other ingredients except lettuce leaves. Marinate for at least 30 minutes in the refrigerator.

Stir-fry meat in a pan until it is cooked. Serve with rice and lettuce leaves. Wrap rice and meat with a piece of lettuce leaf and enjoy.

Per serving: 336 calories, 23 g fat (7 g saturated fat), 22 g protein, 8 g carbohydrates, 1 g dietary fiber.

Fish with Black Bean Sauce

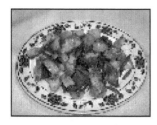

Servings: 4
Pan-fried fish cooked with vegetable in salty black bean sauce. You can also use squid or clam in place of the fish.

1 pound fish fillet, cut into bite-size pieces
2 tablespoons cornstarch
½ teaspoon salt
1 green pepper or vegetable of your choice, cut into bite-size pieces
4 tablespoons vegetable oil
1 onion, cut into 1-inch cubes
1 tablespoon black bean sauce
3 tablespoons water

Sprinkle salt and cornstarch on top of the sliced fish.

Heat 3 tbsp. oil in a pan. Drop the fish pieces into the pan. Cook for 5 minutes then turn gently to the other side. After both sides are browned put fried fish on the serving plate.

Heat 1 tbsp. oil in the pan, stir-fry onion and green pepper for 1 minute. Add black bean sauce and 3 tbsp. of water, continue to cook for another minute, then pour onto the fish.

Per serving: 252 calories, 15 g fat (2 g saturated fat), 21 g protein, 8 g carbohydrates, 1 g dietary fiber.

Salmon in Tomato Sauce

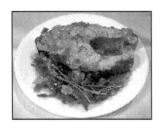

Servings: 4
Salmon in grilled onion, garlic, tomato and peanut butter sauce. You can prepare any kind of boneless fish steak or fillet this way.

1 pound salmon steak or fillet
2 tablespoons lime juice or vinegar
1 tablespoon salt
2 tablespoon vegetable oil
1 medium onion, minced
1 tablespoon minced garlic
1 medium tomato, minced
1 teaspoon chili sauce, optional
¼ cup water
1 tablespoon peanut butter
5 kaffir lime leaves torn into halves, optional
1 teaspoon sugar

Marinate fish with lime juice and salt for 5 minutes.

Heat oil in the pan and stir-fry onion and garlic for 2 minutes. Add tomato, chili sauce, salmon and water.

Add peanut butter, kaffir lime leaves and sugar. Simmer in medium heat for 10 minutes or until the fish is cooked. Serve.

Per serving: 242 calories, 13 g fat (2 g saturated fat), 24 g protein, 7 g carbohydrates, 1 g dietary fiber.

Fish with Soy Sauce

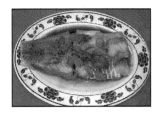

Servings: 4
Fish in a fragrant mix of sesame oil and soy sauce.

1 pound sole/bass/while fish fillet, cleaned
1 tablespoon ginger, sliced thin
4 tablespoons soy sauce
1 tablespoon vegetable oil
1 teaspoon sesame oil
¼ cup cilantro leaves, optional

Put the fish on a microwave-safe plate. Place ginger slices on top of the fish. Cover and microwave on high heat for 2 minutes. If there is some water on the plate, drain it.

Mix soy sauce, vegetable oil and sesame oil in a micro-wave-safe bowl. Heat the mixture for 30 seconds in the microwave, then pour them on top of the fish. Garnish with cilantro sprigs and serve with steamed rice.

Per serving: 158 calories, 6 g fat (1 g saturated fat), 22 g protein, 3 g carbohydrates, 0 g dietary fiber.

Singapore Chili Crabs or Lobster

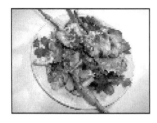

Servings: 4
Crab or lobster in a spicy sweet and sour sauce.

2 pounds lobster or crab, boiled and cut into large chunks
2 tablespoons vegetable oil
4 teaspoons minced garlic
1 teaspoon minced ginger
2 stalks green onions, chopped

Sauce:
1 tablespoon chili sauce or red pepper flakes
3 tablespoons ketchup
2 tablespoons sugar
1 tablespoon cornstarch
½ tablespoon vinegar
1 tablespoon soy sauce
2 egg whites
½ teaspoon salt
1 cup water

In a small bowl, mix all the sauce ingredients.

Heat oil in the pan. Stir-fry garlic, ginger and green onions for 1 minute. Add the sauce mixture and cooked crab or lobster. Simmer for 5–10 minutes until the sauce thickens. Serve.

Per serving: 332 calories, 9 g fat (1 g saturated fat), 45 g protein, 16 g carbohydrates, 1 g dietary fiber.

Shrimp in Lobster Sauce

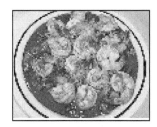

Servings: 4
You don't need a lobster for this recipe. It is called lobster sauce because traditionally lobster is prepared this way. You can also use crab legs instead of shrimp.

1 pound shrimp, peeled and deveined
2 tablespoons oyster sauce
½ cup water
1 tablespoon cornstarch
1 teaspoon vegetable oil
1 teaspoon minced garlic
1 teaspoon minced ginger
½ pound ground pork
1 tablespoon black bean sauce
1 teaspoon chili sauce, optional
2 tablespoons chopped green onions, to garnish

Combine oyster sauce, water and cornstarch in a small bowl; mix well.

Heat oil in the pan. Stir-fry garlic, ginger and ground pork for 2 minutes. Add black bean sauce, chili sauce and shrimp.

Add the oyster sauce solution and bring to a boil. Garnish with green onions and serve.

Per serving: 296 calories, 15 g fat (5 g saturated fat), 33 g protein, 4 g carbohydrates, 0 g dietary fiber.

Grilled Fish

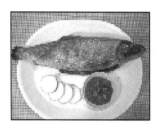

Servings: 4
This simple grilled fish is usu-
ally eaten with a condiment.
Choose between the soy sauce
or tomato sauce recipes on the
following page. Or enjoy it with
salsa or tabasco sauce.

2 pounds fish (bass/bonito/trout/red snapper)
2 tablespoons lime juice or vinegar
1 tablespoon salt
1 teaspoon vegetable oil

Sprinkle fish with lime juice and salt. Marinate for 10 minutes.

Brush oil to prevent fish from sticking and broil it in a pan or on a grill for about 5–10 minutes on each side or until golden brown. Serve with your favorite low-fat condiment.

Per serving: 271 calories, 10 g fat (2 g saturated fat), 43 g protein, 1 g carbohydrate, 0 g dietary fiber.

Soy Sauce Condiment

Servings: 4
This soy sauce condiment complements grilled or fried meat, tofu and seafood dishes. If you like sweet sauce, add 1 tablespoon brown sugar to the recipe.

2 tablespoons soy sauce
1 teaspoon garlic
1 teaspoon chili sauce, optional
½ teaspoon lime juice or vinegar

Mix all the ingredients and serve.

Per serving: 6 calories, 0 g fat (0 g saturated fat), 1 g protein, 1 g carbohydrate, 0 g dietary fiber.

Tomato Sauce Condiment

Servings: 4
This condiment complements grilled or fried seafood. You can reduce or skip the chili sauce if you don't like spicy food.

2 medium tomatoes, chopped
1 teaspoon chili sauce or 2 small chiles, chopped
2 tablespoons chopped onions
1½ teaspoons salt
2 teaspoons lime juice or vinegar

Mix all the ingredients to form a thick sauce and serve.

Per serving: 16 calories, 0 g fat (0 g saturated fat), 1 g protein, 4 g carbohydrates, 1 g dietary fiber

Ma Po Tofu

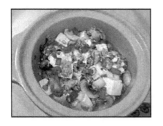

Servings: 4
Tofu with minced pork and mushroom in a fragrant soy sauce mix.

½ cup chicken broth
3 tablespoons soy sauce
1 tablespoon cornstarch
2 tablespoons dry sherry or rice wine
1 teaspoon vegetable oil
2 stalks green onions, chopped
1 teaspoon minced garlic
1 teaspoon minced ginger
½ pound ground pork
½ pound mushroom, sliced
1 pound tofu, cut into ½-inch cubes

Combine chicken broth, soy sauce, cornstarch and dry sherry in a small bowl. Mix well.

Heat oil in the wok/pan. Stir-fry green onions, garlic and ginger for about 15 seconds. Add ground pork and continue to stir-fry for a few minutes until it is cooked.

Add mushrooms, tofu and soy sauce mixture. Stir gently to avoid lumps and cook for about 5 minutes until the mixture is thickened. Serve.

Per serving: 292 calories, 19 g fat (5 g saturated fat), 21 g protein, 9 g carbohydrates, 2 g dietary fiber.

Egg Fu Yung with Sweet and Sour Sauce

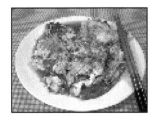

Servings: 4
Chinese-style omelette with meat and bean sprouts, served with sweet and sour sauce.

3 large eggs
1 teaspoon salt
¼ teaspoon pepper
4 ounces cooked shrimp/crab/sliced chicken meat
1 cup bean sprouts
½ cup onion, sliced thin
3 tablespoons vegetable oil

Sweet and Sour Sauce:
1 tablespoon cornstarch
1 cup water
4 tablespoons ketchup
4 tablespoons sugar
1 tablespoon vinegar

In a bowl: beat eggs with a fork, then add the remaining ingredients.

Heat oil in the pan, add egg mixture to form small patties. Cook for a few minutes and serve with sweet and sour sauce.

Sauce: Mix all the ingredients well and boil in a pan to form a thick sauce.

Per serving: 255 calories, 14 g fat (2 g saturated fat), 11 g protein, 22 g carbohydrates, 1 g dietary fiber.

IV. Vegetable Dishes

Mixed Vegetables Stir Fry

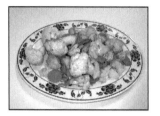

Servings: 4
Vegetables in fragrant garlic and soy sauce mix. You can add shrimp, fish fillet or scallops to make a complete main dish.

2 tablespoons soy sauce
½ teaspoon salt
2 tablespoons cornstarch
½ cup water
1 tablespoon vegetable oil
1 stalk green onion, chopped
1 tablespoon minced garlic
1 carrot, sliced thin
8 ounces cabbage, cut into 1-inch slices
8 ounces cauliflower, cut into bite-size pieces
8 ounces sliced mushrooms

Mix soy sauce, salt, cornstarch and water in a small bowl.

Heat oil in the pan. Stir-fry green onions and garlic for 1 minute. Add carrot, cabbage, cauliflower and mushrooms.

Stir in the cornstarch solution and simmer for 5 minutes. Serve.

Per serving: 94 calories, 4 g fat (0 g saturated fat), 4 g protein, 13 g carbohydrates, 4 g dietary fiber.

Indonesian Salad with Peanut Sauce Dressing (Gado Gado)

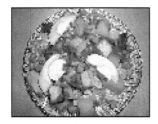

Servings: 4
Salad greens with potatoes, fried tofu and egg in peanut sauce dressing (recipe on page 132).

12 ounces firm tofu, drained and cut into 1-inch cubes
½ teaspoon salt
3 tablespoons vegetable oil
2 medium potatoes, peeled and cut into 1-inch cubes
5 ounces bean sprouts
½ pound green leaf lettuce or mixed salad greens of
   your choice
1 cup corn
2 eggs, hard-boiled, peeled and sliced ¼ inch thick

Dry tofu by wrapping it in a paper towel. Heat oil in a pan and fry tofu until golden brown. Remove from oil, sprinkle with salt and set aside.

Boil potato cubes for 10 minutes or until soft. Add bean sprouts, boil for 2 more minutes and drained.

Mix tofu and potato mixture with remaining ingredients and put in a serving platter. Garnish with egg slices.

Serve salad using peanut sauce as the salad dressing.

Per serving: 288 calories, 17 g fat (3 g saturated fat), 14 g protein, 24 g carbohydrates, 4 g dietary fiber.

Bok Choy with Oyster Sauce

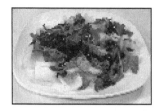

Servings: 4
This simple dish is ready in less than five minutes. It shows the convenience of having a bottle of oyster sauce in your kitchen.

1 pound bok choy or vegetable of your choice, cut into 1-inch pieces
2 tablespoons oyster sauce

Wash and drain bok choy. Boil it or cook in the microwave for about 2–4 minutes, watching closely to prevent overcooking.

Pour oyster sauce on top of the cooked bok choy for a warm, low-calorie vegetable dish.

Per serving: 16 calories, 0 g fat (0 g saturated fat), 2 g protein, 3 g carbohydrates, 1 g dietary fiber.

Stir-Fried Bean Sprouts

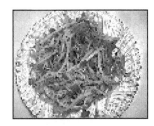

Servings: 4
Crunchy bean sprouts in a
fragrant soy sauce mix.

1 pound bean sprouts
1 carrot, sliced thin
1 teaspoon minced garlic
1 tablespoon dry sherry or cooking wine
2 tablespoons soy sauce
¼ teaspoon sesame oil
1 tablespoon vegetable oil
¼ teaspoon salt
pepper to taste

Heat oil and stir-fry garlic for 1 minute. Add carrot and continue to stir-fry for 3 minutes.

Add bean sprouts, salt, pepper, dry sherry, soy sauce, sesame oil and cook for 1-2 minutes. Serve.

Per serving: 85 calories, 4 g fat (0 g saturated fat), 4 g protein, 10 g carbohydrates, 3 g dietary fiber.

Eggplant and Shrimp in Tomato Sauce

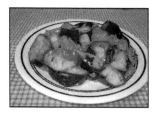

Servings: 4
Eggplant and shrimp stir-fried with tomato, chili (optional), garlic and onion.

1 large eggplant, cut into bite-size pieces
1 teaspoon salt
2 tablespoons vegetable oil
1 tablespoon minced garlic
½ medium onion, minced
1 tablespoon chili sauce or minced chili pepper, optional
1 medium tomato, chopped
1 tablespoon sugar
½ cup water
8 ounces shrimp, peeled and deveined

Sprinkle salt over eggplant pieces. Cook eggplant in microwave for 6 minutes; set aside.

Heat oil in the pan; stir-fry garlic and onion for 2 minutes.

Add chili sauce, tomato, sugar, water, eggplant and shrimp. Cook for 3 minutes. Serve.

Per serving: 178 calories, 8 g fat (1 g saturated fat), 13 g protein, 14 g carbohydrates, 4 g dietary fiber.

V. Snacks and Desserts

Fresh Fruit Salad (Rujak)

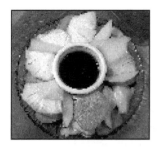

Servings: 4
Tropical fruit salad with peanut and brown sugar dressing.

1 whole pineapple, fresh or canned
1 medium mango
1 medium sweet potato
1 medium apple

Sauce:
6 tablespoons brown sugar
2 tablespoons peanut butter
¾ cup water
1 teaspoon chili sauce, optional

Peel the fruits and slice them into thin, bite-size pieces.

Sauce: Mix the sauce ingredients and simmer over medium heat for 2 minutes or until they form a thick sauce.

Per serving: 245 calories, 5 g fat (1 g saturated fat), 3 g protein, 51 g carbohydrates, 5 g dietary fiber.

Sweet Banana with Coconut Milk

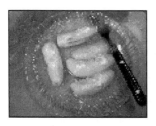

Servings: 4
Sweet banana dessert. Alternatively you can also use cooked yam or mix both yam and sliced banana in the sweet syrup.

2 slightly unripe bananas, peeled, halved lengthwise and horizontally to make 4 pieces
¼ cup water
2 tablespoons sugar
2 tablespoons coconut milk

Boil water and sugar, stir gently. Add bananas and cook for a minute. Put bananas on a serving plate.

Add coconut milk on top of the bananas and serve.

Per serving: 96 calories, 2 g fat (2 g saturated fat), 1 g protein, 20 g carbohydrates, 2 g dietary fiber.

Sweet Green Mung Bean Porridge

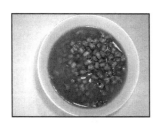

Servings: 4
Serve this porridge warm on a cold day or serve cold with shaved ice or ice cubes on a hot day. You can also serve red kidney beans or black sticky rice this way.

3 ounces mung beans, soaked overnight
3 cups water
½ cup brown sugar
3 tablespoons coconut milk, optional

Boil green beans, water, and sugar for about 25 minutes. Add coconut milk. Serve warm or cold.

Per serving: 168 calories, 3 g fat (2 g saturated fat), 5 g protein, 32 g carbohydrates, 4 g dietary fiber.

Fruit and Shaved Ice

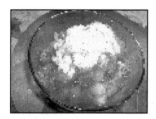

Servings: 4
Mixed fruit with shaved ice. You can combine all kinds of canned, frozen or fresh fruit. Cut fresh fruit to small pieces or use a melon baller.

10 ounces canned fruit cocktail, drained
10 ounces canned kidney beans, drained
4 cups shaved ice
4 tablespoons Hershey strawberry syrup or shaved ice syrup
2 teaspoons sweetened condensed milk

Mix fruit cocktail and kidney beans. Divide into 4 individual serving bowls.

Top the bowl with shaved ice. Sprinkle syrup and condensed milk on top of the ice.

Per serving: 191 calories, 2 g fat (1 g saturated fat), 5 g protein, 41 g carbohydrates, 5 g dietary fiber.

Afterword

I hope this book has provided you with helpful insights and practical knowledge on how to enjoy food and stay slim naturally.

I would like to encourage you with the following analogy. An airplane in flight has a route and a destination. Frequently, while it is flying, the wind pushes it off route. However, the captain keeps bringing it back to the correct path with the help of his knowledge and equipment, so that it arrives at its final destination.

Your weight loss journey might be similar to the plane's path. Don't be discouraged if you catch yourself "off course." Just continue to self-correct using your newly learned knowledge and keep trying to build slimming habits until they become second nature.

Best wishes,

Linda Yo

Endnotes

Chapter 2

"Country Comparison: Obesity - Adult Prevalence Rate." Central Intelligence Agency. Central Intelligence Agency, n.d. Web. 14 Nov. 2014. <https://www.cia.gov/library/publications/the-world-factbook/rankorder/2228rank.html>.

Statistics, National Center For Health. "Summary Health Statistics for U.S. Adults: National Health Interview Survey, 2010." (n.d.): n. pag. Web. 15 Oct. 2014. <http://www.cdc.gov/nchs/data/series /sr_10/sr10_252.pdf>.

Chapter 3

Bilsborough, Shane A., and Timothy C. Crowe. "Low-Carbohydrate Diets: What Are the Potential Short- and Long-Term Health Implications?" Asia Pacific Journal of Clinical Nutrition 2003 : 396–404. Print.

Esfahani, Amin et al. "The Application of the Glycemic Index and Glycemic Load in Weight Loss: A Review of the Clinical Evidence." IUBMB Life 2011 : 7–13.

Bell, Elizabeth A, and Barbara J Rolls. "Energy Density of Foods Affects Energy Intake across Multiple Levels of Fat Content in Lean and Obese Women." The American Journal of Clinical Nutrition 73 .6 (2001): 1010–1018.

Behall, K. M., and J. C. Howe. "Contribution of Fiber and Resistant Starch to Metabolizable Energy." American Journal of Clinical Nutrition. Vol. 62. N. p., 1995. Print.

Willis, Holly J et al. "Greater Satiety Response with Resistant Starch and Corn Bran in Human Subjects." Nutrition research (New York, N.Y.) 29.2 (2009): 100–5. Web. 17 Feb. 2014.

Bodinham, Caroline L, Gary S Frost, and M Denise Robertson. "Acute Ingestion of Resistant Starch Reduces Food Intake in Healthy Adults." The British journal of nutrition 103 (2010): 917–922.

Higgins, Janine a et al. "Resistant Starch and Exercise Independently Attenuate Weight Regain on a High Fat Diet in a Rat Model of Obesity." Nutrition & metabolism 8.1 (2011): 49. Web. 12 Mar. 2014.

Higgins, Janine a. "Resistant Starch: Metabolic Effects and Potential Health Benefits." Journal of AOAC International 87 (2004): 761–8.

Chapter 4

Jordan, H A et al. "Role of Food Characteristics in Behavioral Change and Weight Loss." Journal of the American Dietetic Association 79 (1981): 24–29. Print. Zhu, Yong, and James H Hollis. "Soup Consumption Is Associated with a Lower Dietary Energy Density and a Better Diet Quality in US Adults." The British journal of nutrition (2014): 1–7.

Bertrais, S. et al. "Consumption of Soup and Nutritional Intake in French Adults: Consequences for Nutritional Status." Journal of Human Nutrition and Dietetics 14 (2001): 121–128.

Moreira, Pedro, and Patricia Padrão. "Educational, Economic and Dietary Determinants of Obesity in Portuguese Adults: A Cross-Sectional Study." Eating Behaviors 7 (2006): 220–228.

Kuroda, Motonaka et al. "Frequency of Soup Intake

Is Inversely Associated with Body Mass Index, Waist Circumference, and Waist-to-Hip Ratio, but Not with Other Metabolic Risk Factors in Japanese Men." Journal of the American Dietetic Association 111 (2011): 137–142.

Chapter 5

Atkins, RC. Atkins for Life: The Complete Controlled Carb Program for Permanent Weight Loss and Good Health. New York, NY: St Martins Press; 2004. Print. Dansinger, Michael L et al. Comparison of the Atkins, Ornish, Weight Watchers, and Zone Diets for Weight Loss and Heart Disease Risk Reduction: A Randomized Trial. Vol. 293. N. p., 2005.

Foster, Gary D et al. A Randomized Trial of a Low-Carbohydrate Diet for Obesity. Vol. 348. N. p., 2003. Bilsborough, Shane A., and Timothy C. Crowe. "Low-Carbohydrate Diets: What Are the Potential Short- and Long-Term Health Implications?" Asia Pacific Journal of Clinical Nutrition 2003 : 396–404. Print.

American Heart Association, http://www.heart.org/ HEARTORG/ GettingHealthy/NutritionCenter/High-Protein Diets_UCM_305989_ Article.jsp, retrieved 11/13/2013.

Heart Foundation, http://www.heartfoundation.org. au/ healthy-eating/mums-united/articles/Pages/ dont-diet.aspx , retrieved 11/13/2013.

Food Standards Agency , http://www.nhs.uk/ Livewell/ Goodfood/ Pages/starchy-foods.aspx , retrieved 11/13/2013.

Heart & Stroke Foundation , Nutrition myths – busted!, http://www.heartandstroke.on.ca/site/apps/nlnet/ content2.aspx?c=pvI3IeNWJwE&b=5063573&ct=11633 929&printmode=1 , retrieved 11/13/2013.

Rouhani, M. H. et al. "Is There a Relationship between Red or Processed Meat Intake and Obesity? A Systematic Review and Meta-Analysis of Observational Studies." Obesity Reviews 2014 : 740–748.

Chapter 6

Flood-Obbagy, Julie E., and Barbara J. Rolls. "The Effect of Fruit in Different Forms on Energy Intake and Satiety at a Meal." Appetite 52 (2009): 416–422.

Mattes, Richard D., and Wayne W. Campbell. "Effects of Food Form and Timing of Ingestion on Appetite and Energy Intake in Lean Young Adults and in Young Adults with Obesity." Journal of the American Dietetic Association 109 (2009): 430–437.

Stull, April J. et al. "Liquid and Solid Meal Replacement Products Differentially Affect Postprandial Appetite and Food Intake in Older Adults." Journal of the American Dietetic Association 108 (2008): 1226–1230.

Chapter 7

Hakim, I A, and R B Harris. "Joint Effects of Citrus Peel Use and Black Tea Intake on the Risk of Squamous Cell Carcinoma of the Skin." BMC dermatology 1 (2001): 3. Print.

Jatoi, Aminah et al. "A Phase II Trial of Green Tea in the Treatment of Patients with Androgen Independent Metastatic Prostate Carcinoma." Cancer 97 (2003): 1442–1446.

Jian, Le et al. "Protective Effect of Green Tea against Prostate Cancer: A Case-Control Study in Southeast China." International journal of cancer. Journal international du cancer 108 (2004): 130–135.

Hakim, Iman A et al. "Effect of Increased Tea Con sumption on Oxidative Dna Damage among Smo-kers: A Randomized Controlled Study." J. Nutr. 133 (2003): 3303S–3309.

Sun, Can-Lan et al. "Green Tea, Black Tea and Breast Cancer Risk: A Meta-Analysis of Epidemiological Stu-dies." Carcinogenesis 27 (2006): 1310–1315.

Sueoka, N et al. "A New Function of Green Tea: Preven tion of Lifestyle-Related Diseases." Annals of the New York Academy of Sciences 928 (2001): 274–280.

Su, L Joseph, and Lenore Arab. "Tea Consumption and the Reduced Risk of Colon Cancer -- Results from a National Prospective Cohort Study." Public health nutrition 5 (2002): 419–425.

Hegarty, Verona M., Helen M. May, and Kay Tee Khaw. "Tea Drinking and Bone Mineral Density in Older Women." American Journal of Clinical Nutrition 71 (2000): 1003–1007. Print.

Made in the USA
Lexington, KY
21 July 2017